LAGRANGE PARK PUBLIC LIBR/

SO-AGX-455

3 6086 00187 6082

LP
362.1   Weil, Andrew
WEI
          Why Our Health Matters

LA GRANGE PARK PUBLIC
LIBRARY DISTRICT
555 N. LA GRANGE RD.
LA GRANGE PARK, IL 60526

DEMCO

WHY OUR
HEALTH MATTERS

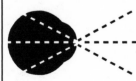This Large Print Book carries the
Seal of Approval of N.A.V.H.

OCT 2009

WHY OUR HEALTH MATTERS

ANDREW WEIL, M.D.

THORNDIKE PRESS
A part of Gale, Cengage Learning

LA GRANGE PARK PUBLIC
LIBRARY DISTRICT

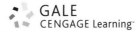 GALE
CENGAGE Learning™

Detroit • New York • San Francisco • New Haven, Conn • Waterville, Maine • London

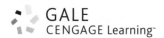
GALE
CENGAGE Learning™

Copyright © Andrew Weil, 2009.
Thorndike Press, a part of Gale, Cengage Learning.

ALL RIGHTS RESERVED
Every effort has been made to ensure that the information contained in this book is complete and accurate. However, neither the publisher nor the author is engaged in rendering professional advice or services to the individual reader. The ideas, procedures, and suggestions contained in this book are not intended as a substitute for consulting with your physician. All matters regarding your health require medical supervision. Neither the author nor the publisher shall be liable or responsible for any loss, injury, or damage allegedly arising from any information or suggestion in this book.
While the author has made every effort to provide accurate telephone numbers and Internet addresses at the time of publication, neither the publisher nor the author assumes any responsibility for errors, or for changes that occur after publication. Further, the publisher does not have any control over and does not assume any responsibility for author or third-party websites or their content.
Thorndike Press® Large Print Basic.
The text of this Large Print edition is unabridged.
Other aspects of the book may vary from the original edition.
Set in 16 pt. Plantin.
Printed on permanent paper.

LIBRARY OF CONGRESS CATALOGING-IN-PUBLICATION DATA

Weil, Andrew.
    Why our health matters : a vision of medicine that can transform our future / by Andrew Weil.
      p. cm.
    Includes bibliographical references.
    ISBN-13: 978-1-4104-2008-4 (hardcover : alk. paper)
    ISBN-10: 1-4104-2008-6 (hardcover : alk. paper)
    1. Health care reform—United States. 2. Medical education—United States. 3. Health insurance—United States. 4. Pharmaceutical industry. 5. Large type books. I. Title.
    RA395.A3443 2009b
    362.1'0425—dc22   2009025784

Published in 2009 by arrangement with Hudson Street Press, a member of Penguin Group (USA) Inc.

Printed in the United States of America
1 2 3 4 5 6 7 13 12 11 10 09

CONTENTS

■ ■ ■ ■

PART I
WHERE WE ARE

■ ■ ■ ■

CHAPTER 1
YOU HAVE A RIGHT TO GOOD HEALTH CARE

"I now understand that when you lose your health, nothing else that you have matters. All you can think about is being well again." That's what a patient of mine said to me recently, a woman in her mid-sixties who was well until a sudden painful illness, an inflammation of bones in her pelvis, disabled her completely and landed her in a hospital. Even with bed rest and aggressive drug treatment, her recovery was slow. For several weeks she lost control of her life, felt helpless and dependent.

It often takes an experience like this to make us realize the paramount importance of health. Without it, the worth of life diminishes.

I have long taught that health is an individual responsibility. It is up to you to learn how to maintain it and to protect your body's potential for self-healing as you go through life. No doctors, no treatments, no

9

system can do this for you or force you to do it on your own. Medical professionals and institutions can help, however, by improving your understanding of health. They can inform you about the influence of lifestyle choices on your risks of disease. They can provide preventive medical services to protect you from common serious conditions — for instance, by immunizing you against infectious illnesses and screening you for forms of cancer that are curable if detected early. They can identify and explain problems that require expert diagnosis and treatment, and then guide you in selecting the best therapy. Usually, the health-care establishment will be there for you if you are a victim of trauma, suffer a heart attack, or need other emergency medical or surgical attention.

I believe strongly and passionately that every American has a right to good health care that is effective, accessible, and affordable, that serves you from infancy through old age, that allows you to go to practitioners and facilities of your choosing, and that offers a broad range of therapeutic options. Your health-care system should also help you stay in optimum health, not just take care of you when you are sick or injured. You should expect and demand this of your country, whether you are rich or poor and whatever the circumstances in which you live. A free democratic society *must* guarantee basic health care to its citizens — all of them — just as it guarantees them basic security and safety. It is in society's interest to do so: The healthier our population, the stronger and more productive we will be as a nation.

Our Declaration of Independence identifies life, liberty, and the pursuit of happiness as inalienable rights of all persons. A stated intent of our Constitution is "to promote the general Welfare." These documents say nothing about the right to good health. Yet, as I've said, without health, life is diminished. Loss of health restricts liberty as much as imprisonment does. Without health, the possibility of happiness is drastically reduced. To enjoy our inalienable rights we must be healthy, which means we must also have access to good health care.

Too many Americans today do not have that. In fact, we do not have a "health-care" system at all. Instead, we have a disease management system that is horribly dysfunctional and getting more so every day. Our health is deteriorating, and we have the highest percentage of uninsured citizens of any democratic society; no other nation comes close. With unemployment rising at an alarming rate, great numbers of Americans are losing their health insurance along with their jobs, further swelling the ranks of the uninsured. This is unacceptable if we want our nation to be a model democratic society.

We used to boast that American medicine was the best in the world, and once upon a time, it was. Today, with limited exceptions, that is no longer true. Even in some of our most prestigious medical centers the quality of care is poor, with nursing services in short supply and hospital-caused illness on the rise. In fact, we are beginning to see a trend toward outsourcing of care to other countries. Our citizens — American citizens — are going to first-class hospitals in Belgium, Thailand, and India for hip replacements, coronary artery bypasses, and reconstructive surgeries. Patients here are dissatisfied, frustrated, and increasingly angry about insufficient attention from doctors in managed care settings, the impersonal nature of medical encounters, and the adversarial attitude of insurers, not to mention the staggering costs of prescription drugs, medical tests and procedures, and hospital services.

I am sure you or people you know have

had disastrous interactions with our so-called health-care system, resulting in physical, emotional, or financial harm. Almost daily I hear medical disaster stories from patients, colleagues, friends, and those I meet when I give talks on the subject. Some have been misdiagnosed and mistreated. Others have come out of hospitals and clinics with more and worse problems than they had when they entered. Still others have been denied health insurance because of common preexisting conditions. The most unlucky ones were denied treatments for life-threatening diseases because insurance companies deemed the treatments "experimental" or "unnecessary." More and more Americans are taking their chances by going without insurance altogether — they simply can't afford it. Without access to primary care physicians, they go to the emergency room instead of a doctor's office.

Doctors, for their part, are dissatisfied, frustrated, and increasingly angry about losing autonomy to corporate bosses and payers. The emotional reward of the therapeutic relationship has dwindled because "the system" has limited the time of patient visits in order to save money. Selection of treatments is dictated by policies of reimbursement, not by practitioner judgment and experience. Many good doctors are leaving the practice of clinical medicine. In the past few years a dismaying number of physicians have told me that they regret their choice of medicine as a career. A recent survey of U.S. primary care providers documents this trend: Nearly 50 percent said they would seriously consider getting out of medicine if they had an alternative. I cannot blame them.

Most people I talk to — patients, doctors, and other health-care providers — feel powerless to do anything to change the cost of health care, its impersonality and the minimal time allowed for visits, or the reimbursement practices of insurers. Most of us feel as if we are up against implacable forces and institutions that are beyond our influence.

You know all this, or most of it. There are plenty of words in print and online that document the medical establishment's dysfunction and accelerating collapse. You don't need me to give you more depressing details, facts, and figures or make you feel more anxious and angry about the colossal mess that is American health care.

What you may not know and what I must emphasize, even if you have heard it before, is that we spend more per capita on health care than any other nation in the world — by a long shot. Yet, by virtually every measure of health outcomes, including longevity, infant mortality, fitness, and rates of chronic diseases, we are at or near the bottom compared to other developed countries. We are paying more and more and have less and less to show for it. We are also paying more and more for health insurance plans that cover less and less. The average American family's premiums now exceed the gross annual income of a full-time minimum wage worker.

Costs of medical care have spiraled out of control, rising at such an accelerating rate that they have become a leading cause of personal bankruptcy. (Every thirty seconds someone in America files for bankruptcy in the aftermath of a personal health problem.) Despite a citizenry so clearly in dire need of help, when I listen to talks about health care in America, especially from politicians and candidates for high office, I hear next to nothing about the real causes of the present crisis or the radical changes required to address it. I do not mean "radical" in the political sense — that is, left-leaning solutions such as socialized medicine in which the government runs the show. The word comes from the Latin, *radix,* meaning "root," and only changes that go to the root of the health-care crisis can save us from disaster. Most commentators assume that the root problems are (a) how to give more people access to the present system and (b) how to pay for it. I strongly disagree.

The challenge is not figuring out how to give more people access to this disintegrating system. The challenge is to envision what we can create to replace it. In this book I will give you a picture of the kind of health-care system that America should have and that every citizen should demand. I will focus on medical philosophy and practice, my areas of expertise. I am not an expert on policy or medical economics, and therefore I will not make recommendations in either of those areas. It is the government's job to find the money for the new system, and it should — *must* — recoup the millions of dollars lost to the present system's administrative waste. The government must also end the abuses of those individuals and corporations in the health-care industry that are making outrageous profits while so many Americans cannot afford to buy health insurance or pay their medical bills.

I believe I have a unique perspective on

the problem. I have worked for three decades to promote health, to encourage greater self-reliance and responsibility for well-being, and to transform medical education and medical practice in the ways needed to support a radically new and better health-care system for our country.

It is obvious to me that the root of the crisis is unmanageable costs. Over the past hundred years medical bills have gone up steadily and relentlessly. Worse, the rate of increase has accelerated, especially in the past few decades. Maybe the insane amounts of money that we spend on health care would be justified if they resulted in superior health of Americans, but, as I've said, they do not.

To understand how health care in our country has become the disaster it is today, just follow the money as it makes its way to the big health insurers, manufacturers of pharmaceuticals and medical devices, and for-profit hospitals, and into the pockets of their breathtakingly overpaid executives. If we cannot contain these costs and stop their accelerating rise, there will be no solution to the crisis and no hope of avoiding catastrophe. The best superficial fixes will merely postpone the inevitable. Even an efficient and fair system of national not-for-profit health insurance for all Americans will eventually be taken down by unmanageable costs. (Runaway costs will also sink the health-care systems of other countries, even those that now seem to be faring better than ours — Canada, the United Kingdom, and Japan, to name a few. Sooner or later the crisis that has brought American health care to its present sad state will engulf all developed countries.)

Why is health care so expensive?

I have two answers to that question:

First, because we give little more than lip service to the prevention of disease and the promotion of health, the whole industry of health care is geared toward *intervention* in established disease — much of it preventable. "An ounce of prevention is worth a pound of cure" is more than a cliché; it is a profound truth that translates directly into dollars spent.

Second, the kinds of interventions that the present system favors are expensive because they depend on costly technology. The Congressional Budget Office reports that 50 percent of recent increases in the cost of health care are attributable to the introduction of new technology. (I include pharmaceutical drugs in the category of treatments dependent on expensive technology.)

Our long-term goal must be to shift our health-care efforts from *disease intervention* to *health promotion* and *disease prevention*. That does not mean withholding treatment from those who need it. My concept of prevention goes well beyond immunization, sanitation, and diagnostic screenings. *I am suggesting that the time has come for a new paradigm of preventive medicine and a society-wide effort to educate our citizens about health and self care.* This must include the creation of incentives and disincentives to encourage people to make better lifestyle choices, better in that they reduce risks of the chronic diseases that now absorb so many of our health-care dollars. I realize that this is a tall order, requiring that the government, private sector, and individuals all pull together and move in the same direction, but it must be done.

Breaking dependence on costly high-tech medical interventions will necessitate making fundamental changes in medical education and practice as well as rethinking the nature of health and healing, the role of treatment, and our expectations of medicine. Without a transformation of medicine we cannot have the health care we so desperately need: health care that is effective, serves everyone, and does not bankrupt us individually or collectively. It can happen. It is happening. I lead an effort at the University of Arizona to train doctors in "integrative medicine," which values low-tech methods such as dietary change, exercise, breath control, and stress management as alternatives to outrageously priced pharmaceutical drugs. In fact, my work to advance this new field has provided part of the inspiration to write this book, because its early success makes me absolutely certain that it is key to getting American health care back on course.

My two main objectives in writing this book are to convince readers that we must:

1. Change the focus of health care in this country from disease management to prevention and health promotion.
2. Minimize interventional medicine's dependence on expensive technology.

By taking these two fundamental actions I am certain that we will stop and then reverse the relentless rise of the cost of health care that has caused all the trouble.

It is the *radix* — the root problem that must be addressed.

To get you to share my vision, it is my job to convince you that these steps are essential for our welfare. Then I will call on doctors, allied health professionals, corporate America, and you — the citizen-consumer-patient — to join the effort to fix the system.

THE THREE MAJOR MYTHS OF AMERICAN HEALTH CARE

As a first step I would ask you to question a few powerful myths that support the massive enterprise of disease management that must be replaced.

Myth #1: Because America has the most expensive health care in the world, it must have the best.

Reality: The World Health Organization recently rated America thirty-seventh in health outcomes, on a par with Serbia.

Myth #2: Our medical technology is our greatest single asset.

Reality: We have powerful technology, but we misuse it and overuse it, driving

21

up costs and worsening health outcomes.

Myth #3: Our medical schools and research facilities excel at creating the world's finest physicians and most productive medical investigators.

Reality: Our medical and scientific infrastructure is extensive, but it is controlled by an almost fundamentalist orthodoxy that limits our ability to understand and promote health and to prevent disease. Medical education today omits whole subject areas of great relevance to those ends, including nutrition, mind/body interactions, and environmental effects on health. We train researchers to think simplistically and focus narrowly on single interventions directed at the physical body, especially pharmaceutical drugs. (The manufacturers of those drugs strongly influence researchers, practitioners, and the journals that report research results.)

I will discuss the power of these myths and my suggestions for moving beyond them in the following chapter.

CHAPTER 2
EXPOSING THE MYTHS OF AMERICAN HEALTH CARE

MOVING BEYOND MYTH #1:
WE MUST FACE THE PAINFUL TRUTH

The *New York Times* noted the following in 2007: "Many Americans are under the delusion that we have 'the best health care system in the world,' as President Bush sees it, or provide the 'best medical care in the world,' as Rudolph Giuliani declared last week. . . . But the disturbing truth is that this country lags well behind other advanced nations in delivering timely and effective care. . . . Despite our poor showing in many international comparisons, it is doubtful that many Americans, faced with a life-threatening illness, would rather be treated elsewhere."

If we do not throw off the delusion that we have the best medicine and health care in the world, we will never be able to change what we actually have.

Here is the reality:

- The most recent World Health Organization rating of health systems, in 2000, placed the United States near the very bottom of the top forty nations, after Colombia, Chile, Costa Rica, and Dominica, and just ahead of Slovenia, Cuba, and Croatia.
- In a ranking of developed countries by the Centers for Disease Control and Prevention, America was rated twenty-ninth in infant mortality, tying Slovakia and Poland, but lagging behind Cuba. One in every 142 American babies dies at birth — more than twice as many as in Japan — and twenty-eight thousand die each year before their first birthday.
- In the same ranking of developed countries, the United States placed near the bottom in life expectancy among people at age sixty.
- In an eight-country ranking, the United States came in last in years of potential life lost to circulatory diseases, respiratory diseases, and diabetes, and had the second highest death rate from bronchitis, asthma, and emphysema.
- Approximately three-fourths of all Americans die from preventable de-

generative diseases, including cardio-vascular disease, cancer, and diabetes. The incidence of cancer has risen since 1975, not decreased, and the incidence of heart disease in females is rising. Eight percent of all Americans have diabetes, a disease that increased by 14 percent in the period of 2005 to 2007.

- The survival rates for several cancers have increased only slightly over recent years. The overall five-year survival rates are approximately 15 percent or less for cancers of the lung, liver, pancreas, and esophagus, and the ten-year survival rates for these cancers are notably lower. Survival with lung cancer, the leading cause of cancer death in both men and women, has improved by less than one month among elderly patients, despite annual treatment expenditures of almost $5 billion. In some cancers, including the type of brain cancer suffered by Senator Edward Kennedy, there has been no improvement in survival at all.

- Approximately one in five Americans has arthritis, the country's leading cause of disability.

- America's obesity rate is the worst in

25

LA GRANGE PARK PUBLIC LIBRARY DISTRICT

the world and is almost universally believed to be a major predictor of future illness, particularly diseases that are most difficult and costly to manage: diabetes, cardiovascular disease, and cancer.

This epidemic of largely preventable illness is catastrophic. The fact that so many Americans are losing not only their health to these illnesses but also their life savings is a national disgrace.

What We Do Well

I don't mean to suggest that nothing about American medicine and health care excels. There is much we can be proud of, including ways of helping people, that we will certainly want to retain in any new system.

For example, our emergency medicine and trauma care may well be the world's best. We regularly save the lives of many who suffer heart attacks and other medical calamities that were often fatal when I was growing up. We can rescue victims of accidents who once would have had no chance of survival.

We have discovered and made available effective treatments for diabetes, hypertension, HIV/AIDS, and other serious diseases formerly beyond our ability to control. We are able to manage many cases of breast cancer as forms of chronic disease that women can live with. We have excellent surgeons and operating facilities where procedures that once required opening abdomens can now be done with minimal invasion, allowing much faster recovery. We routinely save babies who would have died from complications of birth. We can replace damaged hips with remarkable efficiency and success, giving people disabled by pain and immobility a dramatically improved quality of life.

We also have almost miraculous imaging techniques that can identify problems in their earliest, most treatable stages and facilitate the new, elegant surgical techniques, allowing us to do more than half of our surgeries in clinics, on a outpatient basis.

Our advanced computer technologies also hold great promise. Patients can now easily access information that was once available only to medical professionals. And medical records stored in digital form are quickly retrievable.

Also, American medicine has the best research and educational infrastructure in the world and tremendous human resources, including thousands of bright, young, motivated students who genuinely want to help people and alleviate suffering. Properly directed, our research institutions can likely come up with even more powerful therapies to prevent and treat even the most difficult diseases. For example, work with stem cells is close to providing cures for type-1 diabetes and Parkinson's disease.

Lastly, I would point to hospice care for terminally ill patients as an example of American health care at its finest. It helps to make the final days of millions of patients not only bearable but often comfortable and meaningful.

So much about American medicine is good that it makes the overall failure of our health-care system all the more tragic.

Many Dollars and No Sense

To make American health care truly the best in the world, we must change its financial structure.

Costs of services in our current disease management system are now so high and are going up so fast that our society may never find ways to pay for them, no matter how hard we work or how creative we get.

The average prescription now costs $70, and a hospital room costs up to $1,700 per day. A routine adult visit to an emergency room costs about $700. The average charge for an uncomplicated hospital birth is $8,000 (almost as much as eye surgery for cataract removal and lens insertion). A moderately simple cardiac stress test costs $1,900. If you have a heart attack, you can expect to spend $45,000 to $50,000, but if your heart attack lands you in intensive care, that will cost an extra $850 per day.

Cancer treatment can easily cost uninsured people their life savings or the price of their home. Average initial treatment for common cancers runs about $40,000, with the total cost averaging $375,000, according to the Department of Commerce. Cancer treatment with the newest chemotherapy agents is truly pricey: $2,200 a month for Gleevec (taken indefinitely for forms of leukemia); $3,200 a month for Herceptin (for some breast cancers); $55,000 a year for Avastin (for recurrent breast cancer and certain other cancers); and $100 per pill for a drug that diminishes chemotherapy-induced nausea.

Our health care now consumes approximately one-sixth of the American economy — without producing any tangible product that can circulate or be sold abroad. In 2007 our total spending on health care was $2.3

trillion. That comes to $7,600 for every American man, woman, and child — or more than $30,000 a year for a family of four. This represents 16 percent of our gross domestic product (GDP), more than four times what we spend on national defense. In comparison, the medical costs of France and Canada are each about 9 percent of the French and Canadian GDPs. The cost of American health care is rising so rapidly that it is predicted to reach $4.2 trillion, or 20 percent of our gross domestic product, within six or seven years.

Most of the money you spend on health care does not stay in your local economy, helping to support your neighbors and, eventually, you. Instead, most of it goes to multinational corporations. For example, the U.S. medical device industry generated more than $75 billion in revenues in 2006. There are about twelve thousand medical device companies selling more than eight thousand different types of devices; together they constitute one of the fastest growing high-tech sectors in America, expected to achieve a compound annual growth rate of 9 percent through the year 2013.

As big as that is, the pharmaceutical industry dwarfs it. Big pharma (the collective name for the largest drug companies) is almost ten times bigger. In 2006, spending on pharmaceutical drugs topped $643 billion. About half of that was spent by Americans, the other half by the rest of the world combined. In 2005 the top five U.S. drug companies alone had total sales of $222 billion, and the industry as a whole showed much greater profit margins than all other industries on the Fortune 500 list. *Time* magazine noted that "the pharmaceutical industry is — and has been for years — the most profitable of all businesses in the U.S."

The pharmaceutical industry claims that it needs high profits in order to finance its research and development of new drugs, but the reality is that most pharmaceutical companies spend two to three times as much on marketing and administration as they do on research and development. For example, in one recent year, Warner-Lambert (now merged with Pfizer and known as Pfizer) spent about 46 percent of its total revenue, or about $6 billion, on marketing and administration and only about 10 percent, or approximately $1 billion, on R&D. Part of those administrative costs went to CEO Melvin R. Goodes, who made $22 million in overall compensation plus another $250 million in unexercised stock options. Although I am singling out only one executive, the fact is that a number of others made even more money than Mr. Goodes that year. Nor is any one corporation significantly more guilty of greed and excess than the others, because most show the same general pattern of earnings and disbursements. The problem is with the pharmaceutical industry as a whole.

The capitalistic free market system often works well and fairly for both buyers and sellers. However, when the products that an industry sells are meant to save lives and relieve suffering, free market forces are easily skewed. If you wanted to buy a Lexus but it was too expensive, you'd probably buy another car or skip the purchase. But if you need a product or a service that will help control your cancer, the seller can demand an unfair price. This is what has happened to America's health care since it became a multi-billion-dollar industry. It operates in a free market run amok.

Most damaging of all, the wealth that has concentrated around big pharma and the other corporate pillars of the medical industry has narrowed our country's concept of what constitutes good medical treatment. It has made far too many Americans believe the myths that prop up our failing health-care system.

As bad as our current situation is, what we are experiencing now is just for starters. We have not yet felt the impact of the aging baby boomers. That demographic bulge, unprecedented in human history, will make the old and the very old an ever larger segment of our society. Old people have more health problems than young people. Many of them suffer from chronic diseases of aging, including cardiovascular disease and cancer. Many others suffer from neurodegenerative conditions such as Parkinson's and Alzheimer's, which are incurable and require costly, long-term treatment. It is estimated that chronic illnesses account for 75 to 80 percent of America's total health-care bill. In another decade, as the baby boomers reach old age, the incidence of those illnesses and the costs of managing them will increase enormously.

Nor have we yet felt the impact on our already collapsing health-care system of another unprecedented change, one occurring at the other end of the age spectrum: an epidemic of childhood obesity entirely of our own making. Everyone knows it's here, but too few people realize what is coming in its wake: a tidal wave of type-2 diabetes. What was until recently called adult-onset diabetes is now striking children as young as seven.

As these diabetic children age, many of them will develop the cardiovascular complications of diabetes, which generally appear ten to fifteen years after diagnosis. We can therefore expect yet *another* epidemic in young people — one of coronary heart disease. It will take its greatest toll on young men (because young women generally enjoy hormonal protection from this form of heart disease). The diagnosis, monitoring, and treatment of coronary heart disease are very costly and will add yet another layer of financial strain. As the number of Americans with diabetes goes up, we will also have to deal with its other complications: blindness, kidney disease, and limb amputations.

Furthermore, recent research reported in the *Journal of Clinical Investigation* strongly suggests that a woman's excess weight gain or elevated blood sugar during pregnancy can damage her developing fetus, predisposing the child to obesity and diabetes. A 2007 study of nine thousand women indicated that children born under these conditions, or children whose mothers had gestational diabetes, were 80 percent to 90 percent more likely to be overweight or obese themselves by age seven. We may therefore be just at the beginning of a generational spiral leading to even more obesity, diabetes, and all the chronic diseases linked to those conditions.

Look at all these trends, and you will be as certain as I am about where they lead: the total collapse of the present health-care system in America. This disaster cannot be prevented with better pills to control blood sugar, or stronger cancer chemotherapies or the increased use of statins to lower cholesterol or more joint replacements, coronary artery bypass surgeries, and organ transplants. The best of our high-tech interventions can only treat the symptoms of the problem but cannot solve it.

We Must Stop Paying for Failure

If any other major industry had functioned as badly as the American disease management industry has, people would have stopped spending their money on it. But this industry has a tremendous advantage over virtually every other business in the country: Most of its costs, for most people, don't come directly out of pocket. Instead, they are covered by insurance.

The outrageousness of medical costs is often obscured by the illusion that they consist mostly of consumers' co-pays, which are often so low as to make services and products seem almost free. Many people consider their out-of-pocket medical bills to be separate from their insurance bills. People also tend to think health insurance is an unavoidable fact of life that we have long been paying dearly for.

All of this is just more of the modern mythology of American medicine. Your insurance bill *is* your medical bill, and health insurance has *not* been around forever. For most of the history of our country people paid all their medical costs out of pocket, and that helped keep costs down. Most people did not have any health insurance until the 1960s when government mandates for it became common, a result both of good intentions as well as the lobbying of the insurance industry.

Now insurance is a major component of the medical-industrial complex. Its costs are often exorbitant and are still rising steadily. The annual premium in 2008 for an employer health plan covering a family of four averaged $12,500 — about as much as an entire year's pay for a person working at minimum wage. In that same year premiums for employer-based health insurance rose by 5 percent, or two times the rate of inflation; for small businesses with fewer than twenty-four employees, premiums rose 6.8 percent.

These high prices have hurt not only workers but also the companies that employ them. Many small businesses struggle to meet their share of employees' insurance premiums and are forced to pay lower wages in order to cover it. Even though large companies can absorb this expense more easily, it is still one of their heaviest financial burdens, resulting in lower pay to workers and higher prices for products and services. For example, Starbucks' chairman Howard Schultz recently noted that his company spends $200 million per year on insurance for its employees — more than the company spends on coffee. He said that increases in insurance costs are "nonsustainable" and that America is "on a collision course" with the rising expense of health care.

And such pricey insurance still doesn't protect a great many people from financial ruin when they get sick. A recent Harvard University study showed that 68 percent of surveyed people who filed for bankruptcy had health insurance, but in spite of it they struggled with an average out-of-pocket medical debt of $12,000. Another study indicated that 1.5 million families lose their homes to foreclosure every year due at least partly to medical bills.

For many people the annual cost of insurance is significantly more than the amount they typically spend in a year at doctors' offices and drugstores. Thus, insurance costs alone, even without any significant medical care attached to them, cause many families to suffer. A study of Iowa consumers, for example, revealed that insurance costs forced 86 percent of people surveyed to cut back on their savings and 44 percent of them to cut back their spending on food and heating. According to the Kaiser Family Foundation, premiums for employer-sponsored health insurance since 1999 have been rising four times faster, on average, than workers' earnings.

Our current system of insurance often puts both doctors and consumers in adversarial roles with insurance companies, and it has also driven a wedge between patients and doctors, who must select treatments based on reimbursement practices rather than on their best judgment.

Patients who are responsible for only small co-pays for services or drugs frequently don't even bother to find out what the full costs are. This allows sellers to charge whatever they want as long as they can get insurance reimbursement, and it encourages patients to be extravagant consumers of health-care products and services, many of them unnecessary. Imagine if consumers did not pay for their groceries out of pocket but just had to come up with a $10 co-pay at the checkout. It is easy to picture what would be in most grocery carts: lobster, steaks, champagne, and other luxuries that should not be everyday items, certainly not in a health-promoting diet.

In short, the current domination of health care by the insurance industry makes many dollars (for a few) but no sense. Here instead is what we need.

A System That Serves the People Who Pay for It

First, we must face a harsh fact: However dysfunctional our health-care system, however poor our health outcomes, however much our quality of care has deteriorated, however many of our citizens are uninsured or underinsured, the American health-care industry creates a lot of jobs and makes a lot of money — and those who benefit from it have no motivation to change it.

It is up to us, therefore, to create a new system, or we will never have one.

The system that I propose — one that is based on disease prevention, health promotion, and integrative medicine — will not be nearly as expensive as the current enterprise of disease management, because it will not operate in a constant crisis mode, always using the most expensive methods available to treat severe forms of disease. There are a number of reasonable options for financing this system, including single payer models, universal coverage, rationed care, and government-run health insurance. One approach that I endorse is to expand the very efficient forty-year-old Medicare system to cover all Americans. Not being a policy expert, I do not know what option will work best, but I am certain that if America spends anywhere close to its current 16 percent of GDP in the right ways, we can easily have the kind of health care we deserve.

I am equally certain that medicine cannot serve people well if it is forced to operate in a predominantly for-profit mode. It may seem as if health care has always been centered around a standard business model of making money, but this is actually a relatively recent phenomenon that dates back just a few decades. It is not necessary for health care to be wildly profitable — or profitable at all — in order to be good. The priorities and motives of those who manage for-profit medical enterprises are fundamentally at odds with those of physicians, patients, and good medical practice. We have been living with for-profit medicine for three decades. It has failed us miserably, and we must give it up. It is a major reason that both patients and doctors are so dissatisfied, frustrated, and angry.

I am also convinced that our health insurance system should not be fiercely profit driven. If it is to remain solely in the private sector, we cannot allow that industry to reap the staggering profits it currently does, especially with American health care on the verge of economic collapse. When the chief objective of insurers is to make a great deal of money — guess what? They will put most of their energy into finding ways to avoid paying for services. Not only will they charge as much as they can, but they will make it their business to restrict coverage and deny claims whenever possible.

The Change We Need

As a physician my highest priority is to get to the root of health problems. The kind of medicine I practice and teach focuses on correcting underlying causes of disease, not just on managing symptoms. *The American health-care system is sick and possibly dying.* Let me diagnose it and treat it as I would a patient.

A patient I saw recently will serve as an

example: a relatively healthy man in his mid-thirties with a very common ailment — gastro-esophageal reflux disorder (GERD) — that gave him burning upper abdominal pain, belching, and uncomfortable regurgitation of acidic stomach contents into his lower esophagus.

This *very* preventable problem, which accounts for 4.6 million doctor visits each year, is a major risk factor for esophageal cancer, one of the most difficult cancers to cure, requiring the most aggressive (and costly) treatments we have. This patient had been prescribed a pharmaceutical drug to block acid production in his stomach, which is the standard conventional treatment. It gave him relief, but whenever he tried to stop taking the medication, the symptoms returned in full force, and he did not like the idea of being dependent on a drug indefinitely.

He told me that the prescribing doctor had not taken a dietary history, had not asked about other aspects of his lifestyle, and had not helped him understand the nature of GERD. Nor did that doctor make the patient aware of the long-term risks of suppressing stomach acid production: interference with the digestion and absorption of nutrients and reduced defenses against infections borne in food and water.

I explained to the patient that many factors contribute to GERD, especially stress and eating patterns. This man took good care of himself, but as I reviewed his lifestyle, a few of his habits caught my attention. He drank some coffee in the morning, not a lot but enough to add to the irritation of the upper end of his GI tract. He was addicted to exercise — very strenuous swimming, biking, and running — which I felt he used to "balance" his other addiction: workaholism. He worked long hours, and his job in the biotech industry required a great deal of time on the computer and cell phone. My intuitive sense was that he was wound up internally and that his internal tension was the root of his GI disturbance. It was preventing his digestive system from functioning normally.

My recommendations were few and simple. I first urged him to discontinue the morning coffee and to drink chamomile tea instead for its stomach-soothing effect. I suggested an herbal remedy to protect the lining of his stomach and esophagus: Deglycyrrhizinated licorice (DGL) is a nontoxic root extract that increases the mucous coating on these tissues. Most important, I taught him to learn to relax internally by practicing a breathing technique that takes no more than a few minutes a day. I told him that after a few weeks of implementing these changes, he could try weaning himself slowly off the acid-blocking drug. He did so with complete success and is no longer bothered by GERD or by the idea of being dependent on a drug that costs $50 a month and is not safe for long-term use.

His treatment also had the important side benefit of teaching him to relieve stress, which can lead to a host of other ailments. He feels more empowered, and this will help him deal with any future health problems. I relate this case history as an example of integrative medicine in action and an illustration of the importance of getting to the root of a problem.

This is the kind of medicine that should be the foundation of American health care.

My diagnosis of our ailing system is easily summarized. The cost of health care is unmanageable because we focus more on disease management than on prevention and health promotion and because we depend on high-tech interventions.

That dependence is maintained by the second myth of American medicine: *Our medical technology is our greatest single asset.* It is not.

MOVING BEYOND MYTH #2:
WE MUST END OUR DEPENDENCE ON MEDICAL TECHNOLOGY

Technology Has Its Limits

The rise of scientific medicine in the last century was accompanied and enabled by the phenomenal progress of technology. The benefits of medical technology are obvious. The problems it has caused, including the ways it has warped medical thinking, are not so obvious. But they are very real.

The dazzling effect of technology is a major reason for the health-care industry's lopsided focus on disease management. Priorities of reimbursement both reflect and exacerbate this imbalance. Insurance pays for procedures and drugs, not for lifestyle counseling. This must change if we are to contain costs.

The Congressional Budget Office has reported that 50 percent of the recent increases in the cost of health care are attributable to the introduction of new technology, including pharmaceutical drugs. Something is very wrong here, because in most sectors of the economy, new technology usually brings costs down.

Although I think our high-tech approaches are overrated and overused, I am not a medical Luddite. Medical technology is terrific when it is used appropriately. I would never hesitate to use it for the management of severe, critical, life-threatening conditions. But we are using it for practically *everything,* and it is costing us far too much — not only in expense but also in harm caused. On top of that, it distracts us from the more important goals of disease prevention and health promotion, and it blinds us to the true nature and source of healing, which is an innate capacity of one's own body.

The various successes of technological medicine have made the concepts of prevention, health promotion, and the simpler modalities of integrative medicine seem lackluster and old-fashioned. Words like the "healing power of nature" sound distinctly out of context in a contemporary health-care facility with its devices, instruments, and drugs. To modern ears they suggest a bygone era when superstition ruled and the light of scientific knowledge was dim. The time-honored concept of treatment as facilitation of an innate process of healing has been replaced by the belief that treatment itself is the cause of healing and of any recovery. Before the explosive development of medical technology, doctors and patients valued more natural, less invasive therapies, even though these therapies sometimes took more time to help the body heal itself. Today, most doctors and patients prefer drastic interventions that give quick results. Admittedly, treatment of disease is much more exciting than ever before — look at the popularity of television shows about hospitals and operating rooms. Who would want to watch shows about doctors discussing diet with patients?

As a rule, conventional high-tech medicine is most appropriate in a crisis. It is effective for the diagnosis and treatment of severe illness and injury, for diseases involving vital organs, and for other dire conditions. On average, however, such cases represent a minority of the health problems that most physicians see — maybe no more than 20 percent. *Therefore, the greatest cost savings we can achieve will come from limiting the use of expensive diagnostic and therapeutic methods to those cases for which they are clearly indicated.* This means not ordering magnetic resonance imaging (MRI) scans as the first means of evaluating knee pain or headache. It means not prescribing anti-depressant drugs to everyone who is sad. It means not sending all patients with coronary insufficiency to operating rooms for angioplasty.

Besides being expensive, high-tech medicine can be risky. For example, X-rays and computed tomography (CT) scans expose the body to ionizing radiation, which increases the risk of cancer. It is speculated that CT scans being done now will result in as many as 2 percent of the fatal cancers that will occur in the next ten to twenty years. Even mammograms can be dangerous. For women who are at high risk for breast cancer (by family history, for example), the risk/benefit ratio of mammograms may be favorable, but for women between forty and forty-nine who do not have a positive family history, risk may overshadow benefit. Nevertheless, the American Cancer Society urges all American women forty or older to have regular mammograms.

Similarly, some doctors promote routine CT scans of the chest to detect early lung cancer, but here the risk/benefit ratio is clearly unfavorable. I have known several lucky individuals who were found to have early, treatable malignant lung tumors on CT scans, but in the absence of symptoms and significant risk factors — particularly smoking — routine CT scans of the chest are potentially more harmful than helpful.

In addition, indiscriminate use of the new

high-tech scanners frequently turns up anomalous findings that have no clinical significance but still draw the attention of doctors, make patients anxious, and lead to more intensive and invasive testing. Patients in these situations are drawn deeper into the world of hospital medicine, where they may be persuaded to accept unnecessary treatments. The end result is even more expense and sometimes grave physical harm. A healthy man in his mid-forties came to me last year in a state of great anxiety because an MRI scan of his brain, inappropriately ordered to evaluate transient dizziness, showed a slight abnormality that the radiologist reported as "probably irrelevant." All other tests, including a complete neurological examination, were normal. The man was convinced he had a brain tumor or some other sort of time bomb in his head and had gone to other specialists. He now wanted further testing "from head to toe," including more brain scans. I had to convince him that his only problem was work-related stress and medically caused anxiety.

As if that is not enough to ponder, consider also that costly diagnostic scans are now a mainstay of "defensive medicine." That is, doctors order them not for medical reasons but to protect themselves from the ever-present threat of malpractice litigation. The percentage of diagnostic X-rays, CT, and MRI scans that fall into this category is high, which is yet another reason for the daunting cost of health care in America. In a sense this is a form of preventive medicine — doctors attempting to prevent lawsuits — but it is hardly one that improves health or health care. Reforming malpractice laws would curb defensive practices and might reduce health-care costs by as much as 10 percent. Although this would not be a radical change (in the sense of getting to the root of our health care crisis), it would be a step in the right direction.

One of the worst aspects of overreliance on technology is the complacency it can create in patients. Dr. Elizabeth Steiner, of Oregon Health & Science University, recently noted, "Now there is a general expectation that we can fix anything with a pill or a procedure. People believe they can live whatever lifestyle they want, and we can wave a magic wand and fix the consequences." Unfortunately, this is exactly what many of the providers of medical technology *want* people to believe. A Dartmouth University study found that medical centers often advertise unproven treatments and suggest to consumers that expensive technology results in better care. When patients use highly promoted new procedures, however, they are four times more likely to be disappointed with the results than are patients who use more traditional treatment, according to a Duke University study.

To boost sales of their products, drug companies now routinely sponsor direct-to-consumer ads on television and in print media. Such advertising has created a number of new overnight sensations — before the products were sufficiently evaluated by America's researchers. The arthritis drug Vioxx is an example. It was marketed directly to consumers so aggressively that 100 million prescriptions were written for it before ten studies revealed that it significantly increased the risk of heart attack. It was then removed from the marketplace. America is one of only two developed countries — New Zealand is the other — which allows this seductive type of advertising that has dangerously warped medical practice.

Technology can work wonders, particularly in a crisis, but it is not the source of health and healing and should not be overused or misused in American health care of the future.

A Less Futuristic Future

We must begin to break our dependence on costly high-tech medical interventions even though it may seem counterintuitive to take a *less* "futuristic" path to the future. To do so, medical professionals must recognize the limitations of technology and apply that understanding to medical education, research, and practice. Also, patients will need to rethink their own beliefs about the nature of health and healing, the role of treatment, and their expectations of medicine. All this can be done. It is being done at a number of progressive medical institutions in America, including the Arizona Center for Integrative Medicine. We train doctors to value low-tech, "high-touch" methods — such as dietary change and breathing exercises — as alternatives to outrageously priced pharmaceutical drugs and other interventions that are much less cost effective. This effort is quickly gaining momentum and is beginning to change medical practice in our country. But its influence on practitioners and the public is still insignificant compared to that of the pharmaceutical industry.

Making professionals aware of the utility and cost-effectiveness of alternative treatments can do little if most patients continue to be infatuated with medical technology and to prefer quick fixes. People need to recognize and have confidence in their own innate power to heal in order to resist the manipulations of direct-to-consumer drug advertising. Only then will they stop demanding faddish new treatments even when their doctors advise against them. They will also need to accept the fact that medical innovation does not always equate with true progress. None of this will be easy, because as the financial climate of health care worsens, the incentive to use new products of medical technology will increase. As Dr. John Santa, director of the *Consumer Reports* Health Ratings Center, said recently, "Everybody stands to make a lot of money using the newest drugs and devices. The whole business model is oriented toward rewarding the new and different."

I would like to see the use of high-tech medicine become a specialty rather than the norm of all practices. Just as trauma management is now concentrated in specialized facilities (Level 1 Trauma Centers) that serve large regions, we might best reserve high-tech medicine for large, specialized hospitals serving major population centers. Common health problems would then be treated elsewhere in more cost-effective ways. Economics will likely drive this trend. Smaller hospitals and rural health centers will simply not be able to afford the most expensive technological hardware; they will either go out of business or be forced to offer a different kind of care, one based on integrative medicine.

To solve the vast majority of medical problems, we do not need a lot of expensive hardware. It is possible — and often easy — to support the body's own capacity for healing by addressing lifestyle issues and by drawing from a vast array of more natural, less invasive, safe, and effective therapies not currently included in the education and training of our health professionals.

That brings us to the third great myth of modern American medicine: *Our medical schools and research facilities excel at creating the world's finest physicians and most productive medical investigators.*

Moving Beyond Myth #3: Changing the Culture of Medicine: Better Education and Training, Better and More Relevant Research

Great Schools, Poor Education

We have many schools that train physicians, nurses, pharmacists, physicians' assistants, and allied health professionals. They have finer facilities, larger staffs, and better trained faculty than comparable institutions elsewhere. Yet the education they deliver is deficient. It omits whole subject areas of critical importance to understanding health and illness, and it fails to train students in ways that are necessary to build a functional system of health care in our country.

We also conduct more medical research and spend more money on it than any other country, though very little of it translates into better health for our people. Our researchers often do not ask the right questions, ignore topics that they should study, and do not help physicians make the practice of medicine more effective, safer, and more cost-effective. Furthermore, the whole enterprise of American medical research is corrupted by the influence of money, much of which comes from the big pharmaceutical companies and manufacturers of medical devices.

Without a transformation of medical education and research, American medicine will not change. Without a transformation of the fundamental content of medicine, any attempt at health-care reform is doomed. Even the most carefully planned national health-care system that covers everyone will be taken down by ever-rising, uncontrollable costs of trying to manage chronic, lifestyle-related diseases with expensive, high-tech interventions.

Our medical schools are temples of orthodoxy where critical examination of new ideas is actually discouraged. Medicine has always been conservative and resistant to change. New ideas and new ways of thinking are accepted more slowly than they are in most other fields. It seems incredible now, but my pharmacology course at Harvard Medical School in 1965 made no mention of the fact that nicotine is addictive and dismissed smoking as a psychological phenomenon of little consequence. Our instructors were largely unconcerned about how we could help patients withdraw from cigarettes — and this was the year *after* the U.S. Surgeon General warned that smoking causes cancer. I was also taught that atherosclerosis — the narrowing of arteries due to the buildup of cholesterol-laden plaque — is irreversible. Now we know it isn't. And I learned that nerve cells in the brain cannot regenerate — that if they are lost, they are lost forever. Also not true. These errors could be blamed solely on the slow pace of medical knowledge, but they are also examples of the enduring indifference of American medical schools to lifestyle influences on health and to the intrinsic regenerative powers of the body. That indifference persists today.

All schools that train health professionals should teach courses on the body's ability to heal, on its array of mechanisms to identify problems and correct them, and on its ability to regenerate and repair itself. None of this is included in today's curriculums. Another glaring omission is nutrition. Approximately 40 percent of all medical schools teach virtually nothing on the subject, and those that do present it more as biochemistry than as practical information about dietary influences on health, ensuring that students will forget the information once they have been tested on it. As a result, most American medical doctors are functionally illiterate about nutrition and are unable to counsel patients about improving their eating habits.

Nor are our doctors trained to be agents of behavioral change, able to address one of the deep roots of our health-care crisis: our failure to prevent disease and promote health. To do so we must teach people about better lifestyle choices and encourage them to incorporate these changes into their daily lives. As part of that effort, doctors must first teach by example. They should exemplify health and model healthy behavior for patients and others. Unfortunately, the experience of medical school and the residency training that follows it make it very difficult for doctors to develop or maintain ways of living that support good health. Our doctors-in-training must go without sleep, eat the dreadful cafeteria food and fast food available in hospitals, and give up regular exercise. They get no instruction in managing the stress they endure and learn to stifle their emotions. Nor are they taught how to inquire about their patients' lifestyles or how to talk to them about making improvements in habits and behavior.

Recently, an overweight patient who came to the Arizona Center for Integrative Medicine told me that he'd gone to his family doctor — who was also overweight — because he had high cholesterol. The doctor recommended a statin drug. The patient told the doctor that he wanted to try lifestyle changes first, but the doctor said he didn't know anything about that. The patient then mentioned that he had heard the Mediterranean diet could help, but the doctor didn't have any information on that, either. So the patient asked for a referral to someone who could offer more help with diet and lifestyle changes. The doctor said he couldn't think of anyone. I can't blame the physician for all this. His medical education was deficient.

It also did not train him to use intuition, one of the most valuable assets in diagnosis. In fact, medical school discourages the use of intuitive knowledge and teaches students to rely on objective data collected by high-tech methods of observing and measuring. Nor are our physicians trained in the art of medicine — in knowing how to develop empathy with patients in order to listen to them, to sense their hopes, fears, and expectations of a medical encounter, and to present treatments to them in ways that will maximize effectiveness and facilitate healing.

Aside from its deficiencies, American medical education is also very costly, and its high price puts terrific pressure on new doctors, most of whom enter the health-care system saddled with debt. In order to get the income they need, they acquiesce to the standard frenzied pace of patient visits — which average seven minutes and generally end with the writing of a prescription. Too many opt to become specialists, who typically make far more than general practitioners or family physicians. Family medicine practitioners may make $175,000, and general internists $204,000, but these sums pale compared to specialists' annual incomes: up to $911,000 for radiologists, $852,000 for orthopedic surgeons, and $1,352,000 for cardiovascular surgeons. America has a glut of specialists and a serious deficiency of generalists. As a result, practice is skewed toward detailed and expensive diagnostic and therapeutic interventions aimed at isolated body systems. Many patients never get the chance to have their various problems and total health evaluated by a physician trained to look at the interrelationships of the body's parts.

If we need any more specialists, it would be those who are members of the American College of Preventive Medicine. Preventive medicine doctors can actually *save* us money, but there are only two thousand of them (compared to forty-five thousand psychiatrists and fifteen thousand dermatologists). Most work for companies that are desperate to cut their health-care costs, and few are in private practice. When was the last time you saw one?

Much Research, Little Relevance

Most medical school deans feel that changes in how they educate future doctors must be guided by research, but the way we conduct research must also change. Too often our investigators ask the wrong questions, fail to ask the ones most relevant to broadening our understanding of health and healing, and clutter the "knowledge base" of medicine with a great deal of data that should never have been collected in the first place. Also, money from the manufacturers of drugs and medical devices contaminates our research and strongly influences the journals that report it. Many worthless and dangerous drugs are marketed in our country, their use backed by clinical trials published in leading journals. The dangerous drug Vioxx might never have been sold to the American people through direct-to-consumer ads if it had been examined objectively by the research panel of the U.S. Food and Drug Administration (FDA) that initially supported its safety and efficacy. After its withdrawal from the marketplace, following an epidemic of adverse reactions, it was reported that ten members of this FDA panel had financial ties to the companies that manufactured Vioxx and related pain-killers. The consequence of this betrayal of the public trust was stunning: as many as sixty thousand people may have died from taking Vioxx, according to an FDA safety expert.

This is just one example of the many conflicts of interest that now cast doubt on the integrity of American medical research. At approximately the same time as the Vioxx scandal, the New York Attorney General's office, commenting on a similar case, stated, "The ability of drug companies to pick and choose the research they provide doctors in support of their products is an outrageous conflict of interest, and puts us all in harm's way."

It is common for research physicians who report their findings to the FDA to hide all this. A recent Health and Human Services study of 118 drug applications showed that 42 percent of the applications lacked complete financial information, and fewer than 1 percent of researchers disclosed possible conflicts of interest.

Many of the new drugs that emerge from

this system are not needed; they are created just to make money. For example, a 2002 study of generic diuretic pills for high blood pressure — which have been used since the 1950s and cost only pennies per day — found that they worked better than newer drugs that were up to twenty times more expensive. A doctor who worked on the study commented, "The pharmaceutical industry ganged up and attacked and discredited the findings."

As recently as the 1980s, the government funded most of the medical research on humans, but today about 80 percent is paid for by the drug companies. More than ten studies indicate that this funding situation commonly results in misinformation reported in medical journals. The editor of the respected British journal *Lancet* recently remarked, "Journals have devolved into information-laundering operations for the pharmaceutical industry," and I would argue that this is worse in America than anywhere else. Partly as a result of the deterioration of American research, the best medical journals are now publishing more studies performed in other countries, particularly in Europe.

Perhaps even more harmful than the obvious cases of financial dishonesty is the intellectual bias that permeates much of the American medical research community. Researchers not only see what they are paid to see but also see what they *expect* to see and what they *want* to see. Senator Tom Harkin of Iowa, who was responsible for creating the Office of Alternative Medicine (now the National Center for Complementary and Alternative Medicine) at the National Institutes of Health (NIH), complains that most of the studies it funds are designed to disprove the value of dietary supplements, herbal remedies, and other unconventional therapies, rather than investigate ways they could be usefully incorporated into mainstream medicine.

All of this has a chilling effect on clinical medicine, particularly with its recent devotion to "evidence-based practice" or evidence-based medicine (EBM). Evidence-based medicine seeks to restrict practice to treatments backed by the "gold standard" of evidence — data collected by randomized, controlled trials with human subjects. Other kinds of evidence are dismissed as having little worth or scientific merit.

Although it might seem that careful gathering of evidence is basic to scientific exploration, good science begins with uncontrolled observation. The personal experience of a physician or a well-documented case report can suggest a hypothesis to be tested formally. Dismissing uncontrolled observations as "anecdotal" and not worthy of attention removes both researchers and clinicians from the raw material of scientific study and limits our understanding of health and illness. In its most extreme expressions, EBM is scientific fundamentalism, analogous to religious fundamentalism in its close-minded, strident campaign to defend orthodoxy against heresy (including complementary, alternative, and integrative medicine). EBM zealots blackball speakers from professional meetings who cannot document their presentations with studies published in "approved" journals and have forced medical journals to reject articles that report findings contrary to the prevailing beliefs of the EBM community. Worst of all, they coerce physicians and health-care facilities into using "evidence-based" interventions, pharmaceutical drugs especially, which are usually more expensive and often riskier than methods that a practitioner of integrative medicine might want to try. Note that most of the dangerous and worthless drugs I mentioned above are all EBM-approved and supported by positive findings in randomized, controlled trials

(RCTs).

Such trials certainly generate evidence, but they have their own limitations. The more the experimental setting is controlled, the less relevance it has to the real world and the individual patient. RCTs are too simplistic. They seek to reduce treatment to single interventions with simple cause-effect relationships to the body. But the human body (I should say the body-mind) is far from simple, and a healing response is rarely achieved with any single extrinsic modality. Even when just one drug or treatment is applied, its ultimate benefit is dependent on the activity of the body's own healing system. When antibiotic therapy rescues a critically ill victim of bacterial pneumonia, it is the immune system that deserves much of the credit. Antibiotics reduce populations of susceptible germs to low enough levels that the immune system is able to take over and finish the job it could not do when it was overwhelmed.

RCTs often blatantly ignore the complexity of the human organism as well as differences among individuals. And they completely disregard and devalue the art of medicine, especially the ways skilled practitioners present treatments to patients to maximize benefit. This kind of research has great difficulty studying the complex interventions that integrative medicine uses. My treatment plans always include recommendations about food choices, dietary supplements, physical activity, mind/body therapies, and more. I want to know how such a complex package of integrative treatment stacks up against conventional treatment for the same condition, in terms of medical effectiveness, cost-effectiveness, and patient satisfaction. It is that kind of evidence we need in order to guide clinical medicine in a direction that better serves individuals and society. It is the kind of evidence that the randomized controlled trials so loved by evidence-based-medicine zealots cannot deliver.

EBM assumes that the practice of medicine is all science when in fact it is both science *and* art. The integrative medicine curriculum at our Arizona center includes instruction in the Art of Medicine so that practitioners can use the findings of scientific research to elicit healing more reliably.

America still has the best infrastructure in the world for medical education and medical research. However, we must demand, at this critically transformative time, that the *content and direction* of our medical education and research be as good as the infrastructure that supports them.

Creating a New Culture of Medicine

To give all American citizens the type of health care that they deserve, we must transform not only the delivery system and content of medicine but also *the culture of American medicine.*

My colleagues and I in Tucson have been working at this since 1994. When I first began to teach integrative medicine, many of my colleagues at the University of Arizona advised me to make research the main focus of our program. They felt that the best way to win over critics was to conduct randomized, controlled trials (RCTs) on various promising but unconventional treatments and to publish the results of these trials. I did not agree. I have learned that in medicine, as in the world at large, people believe what they want to believe, and they refuse to believe what they do not want to believe, no matter how much evidence there is to the contrary. It seemed to me, therefore, that it would be more useful to focus on changing the culture of medicine by training a new generation of practitioners; they would be less likely to reject unfamiliar ideas without even considering them.

I have long known that many physicians,

researchers, and medical school faculty members have personally benefited from unorthodox therapies but are hesitant to discuss them with colleagues due to fear of censure. Many doctors have told me about cases of spontaneous healing that they have witnessed in patients, some correlated with mental or emotional changes. These doctors did not need data from randomized, controlled trials to convince them of the reality of their own experiences. What they needed was assurance that it was acceptable to talk about such experiences with colleagues and allow them to influence their philosophy and style of medical practice.

I set out to build a community of health professionals trained to think differently. I wanted our physician-fellows to learn to study, practice, and teach medicine from an expanded philosophical model, one that emphasizes the organism's innate potential for healing, acknowledges the reality of nonmaterial influences on the physical body, and recognizes the complexity of nature. I also wanted our graduates to be open to the possible value of ideas and practices outside of mainstream medicine, including those from the healing traditions of other cultures. I wanted them to be good scientists — *open-minded skeptics* — willing to consider new and unfamiliar information about health and treatment and be able to evaluate this information by the standards of good research. I expected them to learn to be empathetic, caring people who are skilled in the art of medicine and able to take full advantage of the healing potential of the doctor-patient relationship. And I hoped to see them become exemplars of health and healthy lifestyles.

Currently, the Arizona Center for Integrative Medicine has an active research program and clinic, but our main effort continues to be education. We have produced a new generation of health professionals (not only doctors but also nurse-practitioners, medical students, and residents) who are beginning to influence American medicine. Some of our graduates are academic leaders; some have written integrative medicine textbooks; and some are starting to train others. I am confident that together they will catalyze the much-needed cultural change that will support a radically new system of health care.

This change will include a long-overdue expansion of the medical curriculum to include nutrition, mind/body medicine, environmental and lifestyle influences on health, botanical remedies, dietary supplements, alternative therapies, spirituality, and more. In medical schools of the future, students must have time and incentives to attend to their own well-being so that they can become not only knowledgeable physicians but also good role models of health for their patients.

Transformation of American medical education must occur in conjunction with similar changes in the education and training of nurses, pharmacists, and allied health professionals. All our health professionals must have a much greater understanding of how to prevent disease and promote health, and they must be familiar with all possible therapies, both conventional and unconventional. Certainly, their selection of therapies should be guided by scientific evidence, but I urge practitioners to use a sliding scale of evidence: The greater the potential of a treatment to cause harm, the stricter the standard of evidence it should be held to for efficacy. This way of evaluating treatments is much more useful than focusing narrow-mindedly on the results of RCTs (which all too often encourage the use of expensive drugs and procedures later found to do more harm than good).

We must also produce more medical generalists and fewer specialists. In 1990, 9 percent of graduating medical students planned to work in primary care, and today that number has dropped to just 2 percent. Money certainly accounts for some of the decline. Over a recent nine-year period the incomes of doctors in several of the common specialties rose by 65 percent, to 97 percent, while those of generalists increased by only 21 percent. This gap should be narrowed — by subsidies if necessary.

When we started teaching integrative medicine, individual physicians came to our center, more each year, but very few other medical institutions showed much interest in our model. Not until the late 1990s, when the economics of health care really soured, did the profession at large take notice. Today more than a third of the nation's medical schools are members of the Consortium of Academic Health Centers for Integrative Medicine (www .imconsortium.org). Application to join must come from a dean or chancellor, and the institution must demonstrate commitment to integrative medicine in at least two of their three main areas of activity: teaching, research, and clinical care.

What We Have to Stop Before We Can Start

To make American medical research fulfill its potential in guiding medical practice and supporting a new system of health care, we must first stop the drug companies themselves from funding most of our drug research. We should also prohibit researchers and regulators from receiving gifts, speaking fees, travel fees, and other honorariums from industry.

In addition, we all need to become aware of the limitations of RCTs. These trials can be very useful, but they are not the only way to increase our knowledge of health and illness and are just not appropriate for every investigation. Many issues are too complex to be explored by this approach. In areas where RCTs aren't suitable, we need to rely on careful clinical observation and case studies. The former director of the NIH National Center for Complementary and Alternative Medicine used to open his lectures with a slide that read, "The plural of 'anecdote' is not 'evidence.' " I would change that to "The plural of 'anecdote' is 'hypothesis.' " It is uncontrolled observation that generates ideas to be tested.

And we must begin to organize *effectiveness studies* and *outcome studies* to compare the usefulness and cost of integrative versus conventional medicine in managing common conditions.

Besides changing *how* we research, we need to change *what* we research even if the results won't yield much income for industry. I want the federal government to create a National Institute for Health and Healing at NIH and put a large percentage of its budget into research of the human body's healing system and the mechanisms by which the body maintains equilibrium (homeostasis), defends itself from harm, regenerates lost and damaged tissue, and adapts to injury and loss.

Lack of research of this sort is one reason that the innate healing potential of the human organism is not part of the curriculums of schools of medicine, nursing, and pharmacy. The body's healing system is not an array of organs and structures that can be pictured neatly in a chart, but it is just as real as the digestive system or the nervous system. It is an operating system of the body that depends on the functions of many interrelated organs to maintain internal and external balance. I believe that the body's abilities to self-regulate, to self-diagnose, to repair, and to regenerate are the most marvelous features of our biology. Thorough knowledge of them is essential to becoming a competent health practitioner. It is worse than regrettable that America spends billions of dollars every year on drug research but next to nothing to elucidate our innate healing mechanisms.

Despite the terrible inertia that weighs against change in America's health education and research, I cannot help but be optimistic about our ability to reform these two pivotal institutions. My hope springs from a practical and tangible source: my own experience.

BEYOND THE THREE MYTHS

The primary benefit of discarding these myths and emerging clear-eyed into the real world is that when we do, we will no longer be so passive in our acceptance of the daily absurdities of American health care. The truth, as they say, will set you free.

If we accept the reality that we don't have the best medicine in the world — even though we're paying for the best — we will be able to summon the righteous indignation needed to overturn a system that makes a few of us very rich and is very well entrenched.

If we see that our technology is the prime mover of medical expense rather than improved health, we will be able to find out what really works best and is most cost effective.

And if we at last acknowledge that our medical education and research systems are not serving us well, we will be able to transform them.

In the next few chapters I will continue to describe the new kind of health care that America should have: a system focused on prevention and health promotion and based on the principles and practice of integrative medicine. And I will offer detailed suggestions for what we need to do in order to make this new system a reality.

■ ■ ■ ■

PART II
WHERE WE NEED
TO BE

■ ■ ■ ■

CHAPTER 3
MOVING TO THE FUTURE WHILE LEARNING FROM THE PAST

Imagine that a doctor visit of the future would be like this: A worried mother calls her family doctor and tells his receptionist that her son is sick and needs to be seen. The receptionist offers an appointment for later that same day and adds that for a moderate extra fee the doctor can make a house call if necessary. This would not be difficult, because the physician lives in the neighborhood (and knows the whole family as friends, not just as patients).

No one in this family needs to see the doctor very often, because they all take good care of themselves and know how to treat common ailments with home remedies.

After his last office visit, the doctor makes his house call. The mother offers the doctor a cup of tea as he sits down beside her son. He puts a hand on the boy's forehead and listens to his chest with a stethoscope. His comforting presence immediately makes the boy feel better and the mother less anxious. The illness appears to be a viral upper respiratory infection with a bronchial cough, not requiring prescribed medication. After reassuring the patient and his mother, the physician, in no rush to leave, chats with the mother about simple measures that will ease the boy's symptoms, including a vaporizer for his congestion. It is obvious that the doctor cares about the child. He also loves his profession, makes a good living, and enjoys the respect of the community. For a few minutes he talks about the rewards of a career in medicine, because he knows the boy is interested in becoming a doctor someday.

Two days later the doctor phones the mother to ask about the patient. The boy is already back in school, feeling fine.

This is my vision of medicine of the future — caring, personalized, affordable, not always dependent on medication and technology, safe and effective. It is a form of integrative medicine in practice, medicine that honors the body's capacity for self-healing and supports it, whenever possible, with simple interventions.

THE GOLDEN AGE OF MEDICINE

This is also my remembrance of medicine of the past, because I was the boy in that scenario, and the doctor was our family's general practitioner, Dr. Irv Gerson, who lived three blocks from our row house in northwest Philadelphia. Dr. Gerson, a fine physician, took good care of me and my parents for many years. He was typical of that era's family doctors, who were then the most dominant single force in medicine.

In the 1950s the president of the American Medical Association referred to the family doctor as "the quarterback of the modern medical team." That era has been called the Golden Age of Medicine, because even though most of today's high-tech methods of diagnosis and treatment did not exist, it was a time when average working people could afford excellent health care, were leery of drastic medical intervention, and practiced good health habits, including sound nutrition, regular physical activity, and recreation. As late as 1958 most doctors were family practitioners, and thirteen out of every fourteen made house calls, usually for only a small amount over the normal office visit fee, which was about $3 in most towns and less than $15 in the largest cities. Family practitioners like Dr. Gerson made approximately $8,000 per year ($64,000 in today's dollars). That was twice as much as the average single wage earner made back then, but it was not so much more as to separate doctors from the families they served, particularly if both parents worked outside the home.

My mother and father worked together, running a retail store in Center City. They had health insurance through Blue Cross of Pennsylvania, which covered major medical costs, including hospitalization in the event of catastrophic illness or injury. I remember my father occasionally going to an osteopathic physician for manipulative therapy for back pain; otherwise, we had full confidence in Dr. Gerson and the kind of medicine he practiced. We rarely took prescription drugs. When we did, it was for short-term management of acute problems (such as a course of penicillin for a strep throat or an antihistamine for an allergic reaction). We treated common ailments with inexpensive home remedies, knowing that we would get better without professional help. Our doctor visits were close to the national average of five per year. We paid for routine dental and medical services out of pocket, which was common; 93 percent of America's drug costs back then were paid out of pocket, compared to 25 percent now. With relatively low doctor fees and much less reliance on drugs and technology, America spent only about $8.4 billion on medicine in 1950. Now we are spending $2.3 trillion a year, almost 274 times as much. By contrast, the price of consumer goods and services today has increased by a factor of eight in the same period. This means that the rate of increase in the cost of health care is about 32 times more than the overall rate of inflation.

During my childhood, hospital fees were also reasonable — about $30 per day for a semiprivate room. Most of these fees were also paid out of pocket, and most hospitals were nonprofit institutions.

The only time I was hospitalized was for the removal of my tonsils and adenoids at age three, which I believe was unnecessary. My mother's only hospitalization was during my high school years for a hysterectomy (for uterine fibroids) — also unnecessary. My father was briefly treated in a hospital for a mild heart attack when I was in college.

My father was lucky. Many of our neighbors did not survive first heart attacks. The critical care that is available today in intensive care units did not exist back then, and without effective treatment, mortality from heart attacks was high. Today's high-tech medicine has greatly reduced that risk, but heart disease is still the leading cause of death in America. We are much better at treating the worst consequences of heart disease, but not very good at helping people avoid it. More than 70 million Americans currently have heart disease — that's almost one in four of us — and the president of the American College of Cardiology recently admitted that "we're delaying the disease, but we're not preventing it."

Healthy lifestyle is the key to long-term cardiovascular health. Unfortunately, the dramatic new treatments for blocked coronary arteries and other serious heart problems tend to *decrease* our motivation to improve health habits. Why go to the trouble of eating well and exercising if you can take a pill to lower cholesterol or count on an angioplasty or coronary bypass surgery to save you from cardiac disaster?

In the 1950s and 1960s people were more self-reliant in matters of health. They did not depend so heavily on medications and did not go to doctors unless they were really sick or badly injured. Americans today are much more likely to go to doctors and clinics for help with problems their parents and grandparents would have handled at home.

WHAT WENT WRONG?

Medical progress since the mid-twentieth century has been steady and substantial, which raises several troubling questions. Why has that progress not resulted in better health and better health care in our country? How is it that American health and health care have actually deteriorated as American medicine has advanced? Why don't we have better health outcomes when we are spending more money on our health than ever before? Why are both doctors and patients much more frustrated and angry than they were when I was growing up?

Outbreaks of polio caused panic in more than one summer of my childhood. Treatments for mental illness were few and ineffective. Diagnostic screening for breast and colon cancer was not available. Forms of leukemia and lymphoma that can now be cured were invariably fatal. Nevertheless, during the years of my childhood, before the age of high-tech medicine, the general population was healthier in many ways than it is now. There was much less obesity, for one thing, less diabetes, and less chronic disease caused by those conditions. According to a Johns Hopkins University analysis,

"On most health indicators the U.S. relative performance declined since 1960; on none did it improve."

Most people don't realize that we were not less healthy before health care became the backbreaking expense it is today. For example, we like to believe that our chances of contracting or dying from cancer are much lower than they were in the past, but this is not so. Despite all the billions spent on research, our improvements in cancer detection, and our aggressive and costly treatments, the overall death rate from cancer in 2000 was almost exactly the same as it was in 1971 when President Richard Nixon began a national War on Cancer. In people who are now thirty-five to sixty-four years old, cancer has overtaken heart disease as the leading cause of death.

Clearly, there has been progress. Lung cancer has declined in incidence, mostly due to a decline in smoking. Prostate cancer survival has improved, mostly because we are better at detecting it earlier. Widespread use of colonoscopy has helped reduce death from colon cancer. Breast cancer deaths are also declining, due partly to mammography and partly to much improved treatments. Also, the incidence of hormonally driven breast cancer has declined as hormone replacement therapy (HRT) for women in menopause has gone out of fashion. Death from cervical cancer has also decreased because of better early detection, and it should decline sharply as more women are immunized against the human papillomavirus (HPV) that causes about 70 percent of all cases.

These improvements are significant, but they mostly have to do with early detection, immunization, and the cessation of harmful medical practices (such as the reckless prescribing of HRT) rather than to major medical breakthroughs. Also, the impact of these successes would be dwarfed by real preventive efforts that may include getting more Americans to stop smoking, being sedentary, overeating, and eating too many unhealthy foods and too few foods with cancer-protective properties. This approach is the direction that we must take in order to make the health care of the future better than that of the past. It is affordable, sustainable, and effective to a degree that will never be matched even by the fanciest high-tech interventions.

The rapid development of medical technology in the middle of the last century led many people to expect that American health care would be spectacular by the beginning of the next century, better than anything the world had ever seen. I was one of them. As a young person fascinated by science in the 1950s, I often spent Saturdays at the Franklin Institute in Philadelphia, drawn to interactive exhibits that glorified technology and hinted at the world of tomorrow it would usher in — one free of poverty, hunger, and disease, and with abundant energy to run labor-saving devices that would transform our lives: robotic servants, climate-controlled cities, and, of course, flying cars. When visiting my maternal grand-parents, who had emigrated from the Ukraine before World War I, I thought about the inventions that had so changed their lives: electric lighting, the telephone, radio, airplanes, television, antibiotics. Had any generation ever witnessed such rapid in-novation? With an accelerating pace of invention, what could my generation expect to see? Was there anything science and technology could not do for us? I remember reading an article in a popular magazine about the home of the future; it promised that by 1970 every housewife would have a nuclear-powered vacuum cleaner.

Optimism abounded, but three emerging trends threatened the health care of the near future. Looking back, it seems as if almost

no one realized how much harm they could
do.

THE THREE TOXIC TRENDS
WE MUST REVERSE

One hundred years ago scientific medicine
was just getting started. The major public
health problem was infectious disease.
Typhoid fever, tuberculosis, diphtheria, and
polio claimed the lives of many Americans,
including infants, children, and young
adults. The percentage of adults who lived
to old age was much smaller than it is today.
Most hospitals were voluntary organizations
set up by religious groups or public works
funded by governments. They were not-for-
profit enterprises, and they took care of the
poor, but back then people went to hospitals
to die, not to get better. Surgery was risky
and painful and therefore much less practiced. Patent medicines abounded, many
containing alcohol and narcotics, but doctors had few reliable drugs to count on.

Because medical education was not standardized and often not grounded in science,
many physicians were poorly trained, and a
variety of unorthodox ("irregular") practitioners competed with them. There was no
"industry" of health care in the country,
nor was there health insurance. Some work-

ers in dangerous industries, such as mining, received care from company doctors, mostly surgeons who could treat them on the spot. Some also bought disability insurance, but it didn't help them with medical costs.

By the time of my childhood, many of these problems had been overcome, but new challenges were just beginning to emerge. As I review the evolution of health care in our country over the past century, I see the great impact of three trends that have changed medicine. They were beginning to shape health care when I was a child and have now overwhelmed it. To make the medicine of the future better than the medicine of past, we must reverse them.

- Trend #1: Deterioration of Medical Philosophy and Practice. The first trend has to do with the shadow side of technology — how it has impaired medicine as well as helped it. Technology accounts for much real progress in health care, progress we want to build on. Technology, however, has also hurt health care in many ways. It has made it impersonal, expensive, and often dangerous. It has undermined our spirit of self-reliance and our faith in our body's own ability to heal. It has changed for the worse the philosophy and practice of medicine and the priorities of our health-care system.

- Trend #2: Failure to Provide Health Care for All. The second trend is the divergence of our society's notions of health care from those in other industrialized countries. Because of that divergence we alone have no national health-care system.
- Trend #3: The Growing Influence of Money. The third trend is the darkest cloud that lies over American medicine. It is the transformation of health care into a growth industry that generates and consumes ever greater sums of money, even as our health and our medical services steadily deteriorate. The malignant growth of insurance into a fiercely profit-driven business is one example of this change.

The three major myths of American health care that I wrote about in chapter 1 have evolved to conceal the force of these trends and their destructive effects. It is comfortable to believe that we have the best health care, medical education, and research in the world and not face the hard facts of our decline. These toxic trends have distorted

American medicine. If we do not reverse them, we will never have the health care we deserve.

CHAPTER 4
REVERSING THE
TOXIC TRENDS

REVERSING TREND #1:
THE NEED FOR LOW-TECH,
HIGH-TOUCH MEDICINE

Medicine and technology are now wedded. That marriage has produced many benefits, but what has it cost us?

First, it has been the main driver of the rising cost of health care, and, as I continue to stress, the unmanageable cost of disease management is the immediate cause of our crisis. Before the ascent of technological medicine, doctors were skilled at physical diagnosis. They observed, felt, and listened to patients. Today most diagnosis is done by machines that are expensive to build and operate. One hundred years ago doctors knew that most diseases were self-limited — likely to end by themselves — and that often the most valuable therapy they could provide was the personal attention and reassurance of a knowledgeable and respected expert. This was "high-touch" medicine, as opposed to "high-tech." Doctors of today are more likely to have faith in the power of the drugs they prescribe than in the healing power of nature or the therapeutic relationship. Even worse, infatuation with medical technology has obscured the true source of healing — the innate mechanisms of repair that are rooted in nature and were honored by physicians throughout history until our times.

In fact, until the technological boom of the twentieth century, all great medical theorists and practitioners acknowledged the healing power of nature and considered it their greatest ally in treating the sick and injured. My responsibility as a physician is to facilitate the healing process by removing obstacles to it or by providing it with needed energy and materials. Sometimes I can do that *just* by giving patients my authoritative assurance that they can get better, that healing is possible.

If the tools of modern medicine can support the healing process without causing undue harm, then, yes, I will absolutely use them. But even when high-tech interventions give good results, I know that they work by enabling the body's innate mechanisms of healing to function optimally and that the true source of healing is within us and in nature.

Also, as much as I am dedicated to alleviating illness, I always consider my most important work to be teaching people *how not to get sick in the first place.* I help them understand what it means to be healthy, why maintaining health is so important, and how we can protect and enhance the body's healing potential as we age. The medicine of the future must respect the body's own ability to heal and deemphasize dependence on drugs and medical devices.

The drugs so widely used today are products of medical technology, and they account for a significant portion of today's astronomical health-care costs. They dominate health care so much that the word "medicine" is now synonymous with drugs, but that is not what the word used to mean. It derives from an ancient Indo-European root that denotes "thoughtful action to establish order." (It is also the root of "meditate" and "measure.") How did "thoughtful action" come to mean "drugs?" The new meaning was already in place before science, medicine, and technology began to march in lockstep through the twentieth century, but the booming growth of the pharmaceutical industry and its influence on medical practice in recent decades solidified it and took it to breathtaking new levels.

As late as the 1970s that industry was relatively small, despite the invention in the 1960s of birth control pills and antianxiety agents such as Valium (which quickly became the country's most popular drug). Today far more people take prescribed medication than ever before. For example, at least one million children, mostly boys, take Ritalin and Adderall for attention deficit/hyperactivity disorder (ADHD). Even more people, old and young, take antidepressants, and pharmacists fill more than 35 million prescriptions for sleep medications every year, at a cost of $2.1 billion. An estimated 81 percent of all Americans now take at least one prescribed medication every day. I think it is fair to say that most physicians and most patients today cannot imagine treatment that does not include drugs. One patient recently told me that when she questioned a prescription for painkillers for ongoing discomfort resulting from a difficult viral infection, her physician — perplexed and annoyed — asked her, "If you don't want pills, why are you here?"

Many drugless therapies that were popular and effective in the past are still widely used outside of mainstream medicine, and I believe they should be emphasized in the health care of the future. I have used some of them with great success in my own clinical work, especially lifestyle measures such as dietary change, physical activity, stress management, and mind/body methods such as hypnosis and biofeedback. I have also seen good outcomes in many of the patients I have referred over the years to acupuncturists, practitioners of Chinese medicine, body workers, and energy healers. Millions of people are helped by these approaches, and yet how quaint, how superstitious, and how ignorant all of this looks from the narrow "evidence-based" perspective of modern scientific medicine with its dazzling array of technological hardware. The ascendancy of high-tech medicine has led us to devalue low-tech, high-touch approaches to the treatment of disease. We dismiss all of them as unscientific, weak, and not on a par with drugs and surgery.

Despite their glamour and popularity, technology-based disease interventions may not help us maintain health and live longer as much as good habits can. A recent report from the U.S. Centers for Disease Control and Prevention showed that over the course of the twentieth century, the average American life span increased by more than thirty years. However, medical intervention — including improved treatments for heart attacks, pneumonia, cancer, appendicitis, organ failure, and trauma — accounts for only five years of that increase. The lion's share of the gain is the result of such public health measures as improved sanitation, less polluted workplaces, safer working conditions, immunizations, and the availability of pure food and water. Another recent study, published in the *American Journal of Public Health,* showed that during the 1990s only about one in sixteen thousand Americans had their lives saved or significantly extended by improvements in health-care technology.

Needless to say, the cost differential between low-tech and high-tech interventions is monumental.

At the time of the recent evaluation of American health care by the federal government, author and physician David Newman, M.D., stressed the importance of making not just policy changes but changes in the entire culture and practice of medicine. "If everybody at the ground level believes that prescriptions and procedures are the things we need to make us healthy and well, then it doesn't matter what kind of policy you draft or what kind of system you build," he said. "It's never going to get better. You can make policy changes until you're blue in the face, but if patients and doctors don't change the way they think about medicine, we'll never change medicine. We need doctors and patients to conceive of medicine and health in a totally different way than they have been taught in the last twenty to thirty years."

To achieve greatness in American health care, our medicine needs to return to its roots. It must focus again on the natural healing power of human beings and be willing to test the efficacy and cost-effectiveness of low-tech, high-touch methods to restore health.

REVERSING TREND #2:
MAKING GOOD HEALTH CARE
AVAILABLE TO ALL

The second trend that has harmed American medicine — the lack of an efficient national health-care system — continues to drive the cost of health care up while driving its quality down. This does not make for sustainability.

The examples that America should follow to reform its delivery system and provide health care for all are those of Canada and the industrialized European nations, including Germany, which adopted national health insurance more than one hundred years ago. Today, these countries have national health-care systems that serve their populations reasonably well. In Scandinavia, Germany, France, the United Kingdom, and Canada, people are much happier than we are about health care. Most of them also enjoy better health than we do, with lower rates of obesity and chronic diseases and with greater longevity.

American policy makers must accept the fact that national plans discourage profiteering in health care and make it far more affordable. For example, until 1966, Canadians spent about as much on health care as Americans, but now Canadians (and most Europeans) spend only about half as much as we do. (Americans spend an annual average of $8,160 each, or $32,640 for a family of four.) Yet Canadians go to doctors and hospitals as often as Americans. One reason Canadians get more for their money is that their system is more efficient, with only about half as much money lost to administrative waste as in the United States. The costs of managing our inefficient system, including those run up by insurance companies bickering with doctors and patients, are so out of control that they account for 31 percent of every dollar we spend on health care, much more than in any other country. This is one reason that only 30 percent of Americans who are sick get same-day care, compared to 45 percent of people in the United Kingdom. It is also the reason that the chances of surviving a kidney transplant are 13 percent higher in Canada than in America and that the survival rates for cervical cancer and non-Hodgkins lymphoma are higher in Australia than here. Wasted health-care dollars mean lower quality of care.

The high costs of American medicine not only hurt individual citizens but also put American business at a great disadvantage globally. Ford and General Motors each pay almost $1,500 in health-care costs for every car they make. But Germany's BMW pays only $450, and Japan's Honda pays $150. American workers should know that their companies could pay them much higher wages if so much corporate money wasn't being siphoned off by expensive health care that doesn't even work. Harvard business professor Regina Herzlinger has examined the gradual increase over the past several decades of companies subsidizing their employees' health insurance and has commented, "As time went on, employees tended to forget that their income was being used to buy their health insurance. Increasingly their perception was that health insurance was a freebie. But it was not and it is not."

The high costs of our health care are even starting to put the American medical industry at a disadvantage against global competition, as Americans leave our country to get more affordable and better quality care. For example, one hospital in Bangkok, Thailand, served sixty-five thousand American patients in 2006, including many who needed hip replacements, coronary artery bypass surgery, and other major procedures. It offers care that is as much as 80 percent less expensive and of generally higher quality than what is available here.

Despite the apparent advantages of having a national health plan, the concept has been resisted in America for many years. Why? Part of the reason is that we are a diverse society, and for much of our history, our federal government was highly decentralized, leaving health matters to state and local governments. They, in turn, preferred to pass responsibility on to the private sector or rely on voluntary organizations. Whenever attempts were made to move toward national health care here, powerful forces mobilized in opposition. For example, early in the last century labor unions fought a national health insurance plan, because they said it would "subordinate workers to the state and undermine workers' efforts to resolve their own problems." While trade unions in Europe embraced government-mandated change, their American counterparts remained suspicious of government intrusion. Even after World War II, organized labor in this country continued to oppose a federal health-care plan, preferring private insurance.

Throughout the first half of the twentieth century, American doctors also strongly opposed all proposals for government health insurance. The American Medical Association (AMA) — much more influential then than now — fought tooth and nail against it, always raising the specter of a third party coming between the doctor and the patient, undermining the special relationship between them, and dictating the practice of medicine. European doctors were more easily persuaded that joining a national system of health care was in their best interests. It is painfully ironic that organized medicine's successful fight against national health care in this country is one reason that doctors here have lost almost *all* their autonomy to third-party payers. Those payers now dictate not only what treatments doctors can use but also how many patients they must see per hour and even which patients are "better" to attend to (because their conditions generate more revenue). Abbreviated visits have severely damaged the therapeutic relationship by eliminating the rewards it provided to both patients and doctors. These destructive changes must be undone.

Given how hard physicians once fought to prevent government health insurance, only to end up with the present fragmented, profit-driven mess, today's doctor would be hard-pressed to find a better, more embittering example of the adage "Be careful what you wish for." Annual surveys by the Massachusetts Medical Society have shown that doctors' levels of satisfaction with their profession have declined every year for thirteen years, almost entirely because of insurance and administrative problems.

For many years the insurance industry also opposed a national health-care plan. You do not have to look hard for the reason: the simple fear of losing business to the government. In addition, the pharmaceutical companies, powerfully effective at lobbying for protective legislation, have added their weight to the opposition, because they dread the prospect of government-mandated price controls on their drugs.

Conservative forces within government have also fought a national plan for many decades, always smearing it as socialized medicine. That term was invented by a government public relations consultant named Clem Whitaker in the 1950s, at the height of the anti-communist Cold War. Whitaker said, "All you have to do is give national health insurance a bad name, and you'll have a Devil. America is opposed to socialism, so we're going to name national health insurance 'socialized medicine.'"

When President Harry S Truman proposed a national system, Republican Senator Robert Taft, a powerful conservative, blasted Truman's plan. "I consider it socialism," he said. "It is to my mind the most socialistic measure this Congress has ever had before it." The AMA, working on behalf of the opposition forces, distributed brochures, cartoons, and recorded messages depicting the proposed system as a Soviet-styled nightmare with government agents ordering doctors to move their offices and telling patients where to go.

If you think these tactics ended with the Cold War, think again. Even after the passage of Medicare and Medicaid, opponents of national health care helped block the reform that President Bill Clinton backed. In 2008, Republican presidential candidate Rudolph Giuliani said, "When you hear Democrats in particular talk about single-mandated health care, universal health care, what they're talking about is socialized medicine." Fear-mongering about national health care continues to this day. It is time to stop it.

Opponents would have us believe that countries with national plans have only the vaguest, most antiquated understanding of how to care for the health of their citizens and that their systems are bureaucratic nightmares. These arguments are as tired as they are false. America's system is by far the most paperwork-heavy and expensive to administer. And our ability to deliver the primary care that could significantly help us prevent disease and promote health has been crippled by our emphasis on specialization, which is far more focused on short-term disease management. Other countries are much better at providing primary care. Sorry, but it's true.

The idea that a free democratic society should guarantee all of its citizens access to health care — a firmly established principle

in the other democracies of the world —
has not yet become part of the culture of
the world's oldest democracy. As Americans
we should insist that this be corrected. The
future of our physical and financial health
depends on it.

REVERSING TREND #3:
MAKING MEDICINE AND
INSURANCE AFFORDABLE

In a 1980 article in the *New England Journal
of Medicine,* the former editor in chief of the
journal, Arnold Relman, M.D., coined the
phrase "medical industrial complex," suggested by President Dwight D. Eisenhower's
"military industrial complex." Eisenhower
had warned that the rampant commercial-
ization of national defense would lead to
nothing less than war for the sake of profit,
and Relman feared that "a new investor-
owned industry that was providing health-
care services for profit might reshape . . .
the system itself."

Even this dire prediction was an understatement. The profit structure of American
health care now drives the entire system.
This becomes clear just by looking at the
astonishing and frightening economic
growth of the medical-industrial complex

over the past sixty years. Here is a summary of that growth presented as decade-by-decade annual totals spent on health care, rounded off to the nearest billion.

The Cost of American Health Care
- 1950, $8 billion
- 1960, $27 billion
- 1970, $75 billion
- 1980, $212 billion
- 1989, $604 billion
- 2000, $1.2 trillion (approximate)
- 2009, $2.5 trillion

Estimated Future Growth
- 2012, $3.1 trillion
- 2015, $4 trillion

As you can see, the cost has tripled in most decades and is predicted to almost double again over the next seven to nine years. As I mentioned earlier, the cost of health care has increased to *274 times* what it was in 1950 even though the average cost of all other goods and services has increased only 8 times. In the next seven to nine years the cost of health care will probably go up to *500 times* what it was in 1950 even though the general rate of inflation over that period may be negligible.

These figures are more disturbing when they are applied to American families. On a per-capita basis, Americans spent only $352 per person in 1970. It tripled to $1,072 by 1980. By 1990, $2,752; 2003, $5,711; 2009, $8,160, or over $32,000 for a family of four. If predictions hold, *a family of four, in the next seven to nine years, will spend around $64,000 annually on health care.* This will bankrupt many millions of people. One of every five Americans already has so much medical debt that he or she is paying it off over time.

What we are forced to spend on health care is using up a larger and larger percentage of our annual gross domestic product (the amount we spend on all goods and services). In 1960 health care was only about 5 percent of the GDP; in 1970, 7 percent; 1980, 8.3 percent; 1990, 12 percent; 2009, over 16 percent. If the growth that is predicted actually occurs, in a decade or even less we could be spending 33 percent of GDP on health care, *one-third of the entire American economy.* That would ruin our economy and our society.

There is only one practical measure to keep this from happening. We need to change the *content* of health care, not just its system of delivery. Health care of the future must be based on disease prevention and health promotion, with a strong emphasis on integrative medicine. Nothing else will save us.

Conventional disease intervention is expensive even when it is done properly, and too often it is riddled with waste and extravagance. We must stop wasting money on drugs that don't work. For example, one recent study showed that patients routinely demand unnecessary drugs, such as antibiotics for viral conditions, costing over $2 billion annually. We need to stop ordering expensive drugs for minor conditions such as $1,000 injections to control hives. Dr. Marcia Angell of Harvard Medical School recently noted that "doctors believe the industry propaganda that new drugs are better than old ones and that for every ailment there is a drug. They learn to practice a drug-intensive style of medicine." Pharmaceutical drugs will always have a place in American health care, but they must not dominate the medicine of the future.

In addition, health-care providers need to stop depending so much on medical devices. For example, medical scanning has become a $100-billion-per-year business even though recent studies indicate that 20 percent to 50 percent of these scans should not have been done. Commenting on this excessive scanning, radiology professor Bruce Hillman, M.D., said, "It's all profits," noting that a group of doctors who own a scanner can make an extra $500,000 to $1 million per year. Doctors who own their own scanners order 3.2 times as many scans as those who don't. One unintentional consequence of excessive scanning is that it tends to make patients worry more, not less. One study indicated that the percentage of patients who said they were "worried" about their health increased from 15 percent to 50 percent during the years that frequent scanning became routine.

American medicine also needs to back away from its enchantment with specialists. Sixty percent of all doctors are now specialists, and 75 percent of medical trainees are choosing careers in specialties and subspecialties. The medicine of the future should be centered around integrative generalists, not only to reduce costs but to provide better care.

And hospitals need to once again be nonprofit organizations. In 2006 hospitals and their affiliates accounted for approximately one-half of all medical expenses, or about $1 trillion. Hospitals are America's largest single driver of health-care costs.

Much of this terrible burden of expense comes from for-profit hospitals. It is estimated that about 40 percent of expenditures on health care now go to investor-owned organizations and facilities and that for-profit hospitals charge almost 10 percent more than nonprofits for total hospital expenses per admission. Despite charging more, for-profit hospitals, according to a 2002 study, had a 2 percent higher risk of patient death than nonprofits. Also, a 2009 Dartmouth study indicated that when cities and regions aggressively build more and bigger hospitals, patients tend to pay significantly more and receive more aggressive treatments, with no evidence of benefit. The author of the study, published in the *New England Journal of Medicine,* said, "To slow spending growth, we need policies that encourage high-growth, high-cost regions to behave more like low-growth, low-cost regions."

If all these sensible cost-cutting measures can take effect, our astronomical increases in health care will begin to subside. Even so, high-tech disease intervention will always be expensive. Integrative medicine, emphasizing prevention and health promotion, is the only practical way to contain health-care costs.

A major reason that these drastic increases in cost and waste are allowed to continue is the domination of health care by insurance companies, which offer the illusions that health-care costs consist only of modest co-pays and that insurance premiums are as much the problem of the employer as the employee. In the future, if private health insurance companies are allowed to keep doing business, they must be much more tightly regulated. Today their chief concern is making as much money as they possibly can, not maintaining the health of the American people.

The health insurance industry rakes in staggering profits. In 2006, in a list of most profitable industries, it was twelfth among fifty-one industries rated; in 2007 it was ninth among fifty-two. In 2006 the United Health Group made $4.16 billion in profit, Wellpoint made $3.09 billion, and Cigna made $1.15 billion. Much of this went to executives. In 2004–2005 the CEO of United Health Group received $124.8 million in total compensation (and later resigned over a stock option scandal). The CEO of Aetna made $57 million, and the CEO of Cigna was paid $42 million. There is no historical precedent for this kind of health profiteering through insurance, and nothing like it exists anywhere else in the world.

The concept of insurance goes all the way back to ancient China. Various forms of insurance existed in the Roman Empire and in medieval Europe. Sickness and disability insurance appeared in the late 1800s, but health insurance as we know it today, intended to cover medical expenses, has a much shorter history. It began innocently enough as a nonprofit response to rising medical costs in the late 1920s with the formation of Blue Cross, a network of hospital-sponsored, tax-exempt companies that offered uniform rates to whole communities. Its original intent was to help hospitals get their bills paid. Why did hospitals need help?

In the early 1900s a new kind of hospital proliferated in this country: the private for-profit institution, operated by physicians, singly or in partnership, and by corporations. The motive for entrepreneurs to go into the hospital business was not altruistic; they saw an opportunity to make a lot of money. As scientific medicine moved into hospital settings, changing their image from death houses to treatment centers, possibilities for medical services and interventions multiplied rapidly, attracting investors. The potential for profit was great. Hospital medicine would come to dominate American health care as hospitals grew ever larger. They affiliated with medical schools, developed research and training programs, and finally became the main centers for the delivery of health-care services.

Relentlessly rising medical costs attracted investors but also created problems for them. Shortly before the Great Depression, private hospitals realized they could no longer depend on patients to pay their own bills. Even then the cost of health care was so great that many patients could not afford it. One of the first insurance plans was sponsored by Dallas's Baylor University hospital, which offered public school teachers twenty-one days of hospitalization each year for 50 cents per month. The day it went into effect, a teacher broke her ankle, went to the hospital, and enjoyed treatment that was almost free, even by Depression-era standards.

For-profit life insurance and home owner's insurance companies had long viewed health insurance as too risky, but the success of Blue Cross changed their thinking. The for-profits realized they could outdo "the Blues" by offering lower rates to healthy individuals and to groups. They drew better-risk clients away from Blue Cross, eventually forcing it to abandon uniform rates. By the 1960s more than seven hundred companies were selling health insurance in the United States and raking in lots of money. The advent of relatively widespread health insurance triggered a boom in hospital construction and expansion as well as rapid growth in the pharmaceutical and medical device industries. But this caused even greater increases in the cost of hospital care — so much so that many Americans, particularly the elderly, couldn't afford it. Nor could they afford all the new drugs and high-tech treatments that doctors had come to rely on.

In 1965 Congress enacted Medicare for the elderly and Medicaid for the very poor, two of the most successful social welfare programs in our history. But medical costs kept going up, leading many politicians to call for nationalized health care. Instead, President Nixon was convinced by a Minnesota doctor named Paul Ellwood that these programs could efficiently contain costs by bringing the insurance company and the doctor's office together, under one roof, as a "health maintenance organization" (HMO). Ellwood said that HMO doctors "would have financial incentives to deny medical services to their patient," and that HMOs "would be better at keeping people healthy" and less in need of medical services. Therefore, profits would increase. Ellwood never explained just how these improvements in health would occur. Nixon's private perception of the issue was revealed when White House tapes were released after his resignation. A taped conversation with his chief domestic adviser, John Ehrlichman, included the following exchange. Ehrlichman: "Edgar Kaiser is running his Permanente deal for profit. And the reason he can do it is because the less care they give them, the more money they make." Nixon: "Fine." Congress passed the Health Maintenance Organization Act (HMO Act) in 1973, and many Americans enrolled in the new organizations, attracted by their lower premiums even though they provided fewer services.

With the rampant deregulation of the Reagan administration, federal funding for HMOs ended and, with it, any semblance of government oversight of quality of care. All that mattered was cost and profitability. The government actively encouraged Wall Street to dive in and invest, while advising citizens to be resourceful shoppers when choosing health-care plans. So began the full corporatization of American medicine, with all the unhealthy trends that characterize the system today: paying large sums to lobby politicians, wild profiteering by insurance companies and managed care firms, and compensating executives extravagantly. HMOs and other forms of "managed care" failed to contain medical costs, which continued to rise approximately thirty-two times faster than the rate of general inflation, forcing more and more Americans into the ranks of the uninsured. In the last eight years, health-care premiums have more than doubled.

American health care cannot move in an affordable, effective direction until the three toxic trends that cripple our system are seen for what they are and reversed. We must recognize the limits of high-tech medicine and stop spending a fortune on approaches that don't work. We need to develop a national plan that will give the American people as much power as the corporations that now exploit them. And we should do everything we possibly can to reduce the greed that has made health care America's largest industry.

How sad it is that caring for the health of people is now routinely referred to as an industry. Until the 1970s, medicine was thought of as a social service, a profession, a calling, the "healing art" — never an industry chiefly concerned with profit.

CHAPTER 5
DOCTORS OF
THE FUTURE

The doctors of tomorrow will have to be different from most of those today. They will practice without total dependence on the high-tech wizardry that many people imagine will characterize medicine of the future. We will not be able to perform robotic surgery on everyone who needs an operation or cure all cancers with wonder drugs. Technology (including better drugs) will still have an important place in health care, but it will no more dominate the future of medicine than flying cars will typify the future of transportation.

In the years to come we will want more of our doctors to rely on the human body's ability to heal. I believe this change will happen naturally as our present system of disease management disintegrates under the weight of self-destructive expense and the reality of poor outcomes. Even so, it must be actively encouraged by all of us — physicians, patients, and policy makers — or it might be so long in coming that the healthy, wealthy country we once enjoyed will become an impoverished nation known for the prevalence of illness and unaffordable health care.

CREATING THE FUTURE

"The doctor of the future will give no medicine, but will interest his patients in the care of the human frame, in diet, and in the cause and prevention of disease." That sounds like something I might have said, but it was Thomas Edison who spoke those words in 1902. Edison went on to say, "There were never so many able, active minds at work on the problems of diseases as now, and all their discoveries are tending to the simple truth that you can't improve on nature."

The wisdom of Edison, one of the fathers of the age of technology, holds true today and should guide us to the future. Tomorrow's doctors will differ from most of today's in all four of the most basic aspects of a physician's professional life: his or her personal qualities, education and training, philosophy of treatment, and ways of interacting with the community.

HOW TOMORROW'S DOCTORS
WILL ACT AND INTERACT

Too many patients describe their doctors as not being "people persons." They see doctors as poor communicators who tend to be aloof and mechanical, knowledgeable about science and technology but not very comfortable around the people they serve. These deficiencies undermine quality of care. Understandably, many doctors purposely maintain emotional distance from their patients in order to avoid taking on their anxiety or desperation. They must learn to protect themselves without losing the capacity for empathy, because the healing power of the doctor-patient bond is great and must be nurtured.

The best doctors I've been to stand out in my memory for several reasons. They were all good listeners who paid attention to what I had to say. They were willing to explain their thinking to me and hear any disagreements I had with it. They were competent and confident in their areas of expertise but willing to admit what they didn't know and consider alternative treatment possibilities. They were curious and open to new information. And they were healthy themselves, dedicated, as I am, to good lifestyle choices.

The qualities I appreciate in a doctor are

similar to those that most patients value. The Mayo Clinic recently did a patient survey that asked, "What traits do you want in a doctor?" Here are the seven that the respondents wanted most, with their comments.

How Patients Want Doctors to Be

1. **Confident.** "The doctor's confidence gives me confidence."
2. **Empathetic.** "The doctor tries to understand what I am feeling and experiencing, physically and emotionally, and communicates that understanding to me."
3. **Humane.** "The doctor is caring, compassionate, and kind."
4. **Personal.** "The doctor is interested in me more than just as a patient, interacts with me, and remembers me as an individual."
5. **Forthright.** "The doctor tells me what I need to know in plain language and in a forthright manner."
6. **Respectful.** "The doctor takes my input seriously and works with me."
7. **Thorough.** "The doctor is conscientious and persistent."

Some qualities that I value very much are not on this list, such as **Healthy** — "The doctor exemplifies and models health and health-promoting behavior." Another is **Broadly Knowledgeable** — "The doctor knows all the factors that influence health and all the strategies for treating disease." As I have written, many doctors don't know much about key elements of health care, such as the body's ability to heal itself, dietary and other lifestyle influences on health, and non-drug-based methods of treatment.

Doctors of the future must also be open-minded and intellectually flexible. I came into the world as a curious, questioning person. My early love of plants and later studies of botany strengthened my connection with and respect for nature. My fascination with consciousness led me to notice and investigate mind/body interactions. I began reading about alternative medicine when I was in college and soon began thinking about the healing power of nature. All this was before I entered medical school, where my independent thinking caused friction with some of my instructors. The more I saw conventional medicine in action, the more wary I became of drastic interventions that too often caused harm.

Why are so many of today's doctors not curious? Why are so few out-of-the-box thinkers? Probably, it's because medical school rewards rote learning more than independent thinking. Plus, it's so exhausting that few students have the energy to be curious. Yes, students who want to be good doctors must acquire a lot of factual information, but what's more important is that they learn how to think and understand the basic principles of health and healing.

Another trait that must become more common is self-confidence. Some patients think their doctors are *too* self-confident, because they behave in ways that come across as condescending and arrogant. But truly confident people don't need to act that way. There are two keys to self-confidence: competence and self-awareness. Both require work and come with experience. Part of that work is to "know thyself," because if you don't know yourself, you can never really know other people. A good doctor knows patients as people, not just as diseases or body parts.

THE PRACTICE OF TOMORROW'S DOCTORS

The doctor of the future will practice medicine in fundamentally different ways.

One of the most important shifts will be an increased recognition of patient individuality, a concept now largely ignored. The goal of medicine as it is currently practiced is to develop procedures and drugs that work equally well on all patients, regardless of gender, age, or genetics. It derives from the prevalent belief that all of us are similar biomechanical units that rolled off the same assembly line — a most imperfect conception of human beings that limits conventional medicine's effectiveness.

Instead of just suppressing symptoms with drugs, doctors will have to identify and correct root causes of disease. It is easy to reduce the symptoms of ADHD — attention deficit hyperactivity disorder — by putting kids on stimulants like Ritalin and Adderall, but those symptoms might result from nutritional deficiencies, food sensitivities, toxic exposures, or social and emotional problems. Unless the underlying causes are dealt with, symptoms will continue, prolonging the need for suppressive therapy with its associated risks and costs.

Too often drugs don't even achieve symptom suppression, because there is an enormous range of responses to medications resulting from differences in genotypes, biochemistry, metabolism, and more, but neither medical education nor the information provided by the companies that make and market the drugs makes doctors aware of that reality. For example, the $1-billion-per-year antidepressant drug Paxil, a shorter-acting version of Prozac, helps some people feel calmer, but others, particularly children, experience "paradoxical" effects of agitation, anxiety, and worsening depression that can increase the risk of suicide. A Harvard psychiatrist reported recently that patients on Paxil had eight times the risk of suicide of those taking a placebo. (This and other studies prompted a federal investigation about a corporate cover-up of the risk.)

Only changes in medical education can change the present focus on symptom suppression. That focus is intensified when doctors narrow their training even more by becoming specialists. We already have too many specialists, or more precisely, too few generalists. Between 1997 and 2005, the number of doctors who became primary care physicians decreased by about 50 percent, which means there are only about 1,000 to 2,000 new primary care doctors each year. Only 31 percent of all American doctors are in primary care, compared to about 50 percent in Canada, Germany, and France, and it's a major reason why our medical care is not as good as theirs. A recent study showed that the states in America with the highest ratio of primary care doctors have better health outcomes than the states with more specialists, even after adjusting for other factors, such as age and income.

Many patients come to me after having seen a number of specialists without getting better. Why? Because none of the doctors they consulted had put the whole puzzle together. They had not asked the right questions and did not have enough information about the totality of the person and the problem to solve it. Medical academics are prejudiced against generalists, considering them not as well-trained or as valuable as specialists. They look down especially on general practitioners and family medicine doctors. I have a very different perspective, being a generalist at heart and a GP by training. I can often help patients when specialized medicine has failed them.

We need to elevate the role of generalists in the health care of the future by paying them more. According to the Bureau of Labor Statistics, 75 percent of general practitioners earn $113,480 or more, but the same percentage of obstetricians and gynecologists, who are not even the highest paid specialists, make \$145,600 or more and are granted more prestige. This arbitrary assigning of status and income can't be carried into the future.

BEYOND SIMPLISTIC THINKING

Generalists are better at grasping the complexity of patients and their conditions. Complexity theory, first in physics, then in many other fields of science, has greatly improved our understanding of the natural world. It acknowledges the reality that systems (like stars, weather, and biological evolution) are so complex that it's impossible to know all their details and predict exactly what will happen with them but looks for patterns that help us understand them. Remarkably, the success of new models based in complexity in contemporary science has had very little influence on medicine, which is stuck in simplistic thinking. This is both limiting and ironic, given that the concern of medicine is one of nature's most complex creations, the human organism.

One example of a simplistic medical approach is the overuse of germicides and antibiotics. It ignores the complex interactions between germs and hosts, including their potential to live in balance with each other, and focuses entirely on destroying the former. This strategy has backfired, spurring the development of resistant and more virulent strains of bacteria that now cause us more trouble than ever. Widespread use of these products has also weakened human defenses by reducing our encounters with germs, especially early in life. It is through those encounters that the immune system learns to protect us from serious infections. Moreover, by disrupting the normal flora that inhabit the skin and gut, thoughtless over-reliance on antibiotics and germicides increases our susceptibility to harm from other, more dangerous organisms. And it may further undermine health by denying the body the benefits of some infections.

Yes, I said "benefits." A surprising example is the recent finding that children infected with a virulent strain of *H. pylori* (*Helicobacter,* an organism that lives in the mucous lining of the stomach) are much less likely than others to develop asthma and allergies to pollen and mold. They may also be at much lower risk for GERD (gastro-esophageal reflux disorder). But because *H. pylori* is known to cause peptic ulcers and stomach cancer in adults, it is regarded as a bad germ, always to be eradicated. Martin J. Blaser, M.D., chairman of the Department of Medicine and professor of microbiology at New York University School of Medicine, who has studied *H. pylori* for more than twenty years, has commented on its beneficial properties in a way that excites me: "These properties point toward a much more complex view of the organism, not just as an ulcer-pathogen or cancer-pathogen, but as an organism that has its costs and benefits to us. The relative costs and benefits clearly differ among individuals."

His words suggest a new way of thinking that can transform and energize medicine, particularly preventive medicine, making it a cornerstone of a radically different health-care system. He acknowledges the complexity of life and rejects a linear interpretation of cause and effect. It is not as simple as: Presence of Germ = Infection = Disease. Rather, it is the interaction between germ and host — both of which are complex organisms with individual differences — that determines whether the outcome is harmful, neutral, or beneficial.

Physicist Steven Hawking, Ph.D., once said, "The next century will be the century of complexity." Complexity theory has advanced knowledge in physics, astronomy, and even weather prediction. To be most effective the doctor of the future must acknowledge the complexity of human health and healing.

You might ask, "How can a doctor possibly deal with factors like individuality and complexity in a standard patient visit?" The reality is that everybody with a particular disease does not follow the same course or respond to treatment in the same way. If today's abbreviated medical encounters force doctors to use standardized diagnoses and "one-size-fits-all" treatments, then we must change the form of those visits.

THE PATIENT VISIT OF THE FUTURE

To begin with, the doctor-patient relationship must be protected, supported, and modified. I strongly favor the emerging new model of doctors and patients as partners, with both involved in treatment decisions. The days of authoritarian, paternalistic medicine are over. With so much information about health and illness available on the Internet, many patients today are very well informed. Doctors should regard every patient as capable of understanding medical facts if they are explained clearly. After all, the word "doctor" literally means teacher. The primary role of physicians should be to teach people how to not get sick, how to live in ways that promote health, how to maintain health throughout life, and how to care for themselves as much as possible.

In practicing individualized medicine, however, the doctor must also know when it is useful to assert his or her authority as a trained professional. Sometimes that is the best way to get a patient's attention, encourage behavioral change, and facilitate healing. For example, when I was a young physician, a woman came to me with a rare syndrome resulting from an intestinal tumor that flooded her body with compounds affecting her heart and blood vessels. Her immediate problem was cardiac insufficiency resulting from damaged heart valves. She needed heart surgery quickly, but she was very unwilling to use orthodox medicine, convinced that strenuous yoga practice would save her. I had to challenge her belief with all of my medical authority and persuade her that a high-tech procedure was absolutely necessary. She did have the operation, which bought her time for more comprehensive treatment.

Doctors of the future *must* have more time to spend with patients, especially with new patients. For starters, a visit should not begin after a long wait by the patient. Some waiting time may be unavoidable, but too much often makes patients feel dismissed, as if the doctor's time is valuable and theirs is not. Of course, a visit should be long enough for rapport and partnership to develop. The average seven-minute slot of today clearly doesn't work.

A recent study showed that brevity of doctor visits is a major reason that as many as one-half of all Americans with chronic illnesses are not receiving optimal care. About 24 percent of patients who were surveyed said their doctors did not answer their questions, 27 percent said that doctors didn't make their treatment goals clear, and 50 percent said that doctors didn't ask for their opinions.

So how much time, ideally, should a doctor spend with a patient? I would like see the government mandate a one-hour initial visit, with shorter times for follow-ups. This is the format I've always used and that the doctors I train learn to use. I ask a lot of questions in the first half hour, not just about a patient's complaints and symptoms but about a broad range of topics. I want to get to know the person, get a sense of their lifestyle, their environment, their strengths and weaknesses. That's how I get whole pictures, and it's mostly how I reach my diagnosis. I rely on that information much more than on physical findings or lab tests, which mostly help me to confirm the conclusions I draw from taking a comprehensive history.

Our current managed care system is reluctant to pay for this extra time. But if we eliminate some of the expensive, ill-advised procedures of high-tech medicine, there will be much more money to go around. Physicians' time could also be saved by making better use of nurses and physicians' assistants.

An office visit now almost always ends with the writing of a prescription. I want to see that change. Not only must doctors expand their pharmacopeias to include natural therapeutic agents, such as botanicals, vitamins, minerals, and other remedies that may be cheaper, safer, and more effective than pharmaceutical products, they must expand their treatment plans to include advice about diet, physical activity, stress reduction, and other aspects of lifestyle that influence health. They should also be able to recommend other therapies when appropriate, from Chinese medicine to mind/body interventions such as hypnosis and biofeedback.

The Computerization of Future Practice

Doctors of the future may benefit from information technology, such as increased electronic communication with patients. Hawaii recently became the first state to offer insurance coverage for physician "visits" done online or over the telephone. Members of Blue Cross and Blue Shield pay $10 for a 10-minute consultation, available 24/7, while nonmembers pay $45. Doctors can issue prescriptions if the visit reveals a definitive diagnosis and receive $25 for each "E-visit," which is on par with their general fee schedule. Roy Schoenberg, the CEO of the company that provides the service (American Well), has said, "There are not enough primary care physicians, and this really allows us to capture care opportunities that might otherwise not be met." E-visits are not appropriate for serious conditions, but they can reduce the number of people who go to emergency rooms for routine ailments, particularly during off-hours. We should also experiment with other possibilities to see how well they work and how much time and expense they can save patients and doctors. At the Arizona Center for Integrative Medicine, for instance, we successfully use group visits for nutritional counseling and mind/body therapies.

Another type of technology that can increase efficiency and quality of care is remote monitoring, such as using biosensors that track temperature, pulse, blood pressure, and glucose levels, and transmit data directly to physicians. This can help doctors follow the status of patients and can be integrated into virtual office visits when face-to-face visits are not practical.

Increasingly, patients will be using the Internet to seek medical information. A recent report by Pew Research indicated that each year 50 percent of adults in America use the Internet to search for answers to health problems. Of these, 70 percent said Internet information influenced their health decisions. But only 48 percent said it improved their self-care. Many doctors are wary of Internet information and are uncomfortable dealing with better-informed patients. But they will have to get used to the fact that the Internet has leveled the playing field, making patients today much more knowledgeable than those of the past.

Obviously, we are going to see greater computerization of medical records. President Barack Obama has proposed spending $50 billion on this in order to reduce medical errors, reveal best practices, and empower patients. Only about 20 percent of all doctors now use electronic records, and switching will cost about $124,000 per physician. That could be helpful, but if it just tracks the course of a dysfunctional system, the help will be minimal. We need radical changes in the *content* of our health care, not just better records of its failure.

THE DOCTOR IN THE COMMUNITY

I also want to see tomorrow's doctors — and all allied health professionals — become powerful social and political forces in their communities and in the country. As they disengage from the disease management system and begin to work toward the higher goals of prevention and health promotion, they will realize they can't achieve them if they stay inside hospitals and offices. They'll need to become serious advocates for environmental change, for better agricultural and food policies, and for stronger controls over the things that make Americans sick.

Why aren't more doctors doing this now? The reason is that they are completely untrained in these areas and highly unsophisticated politically. Political action is not in the medical school curriculum. Doctors not only lack information; they don't know how to be effective change agents in our society. Meanwhile, the corporations that profit from disease management most definitely do know how to play politics. Between 2005 and 2009, insurance and pharmaceutical companies donated $2.2 million to the ten federal officials who seemed to have the most power to reform health care or leave it alone. The biggest beneficiaries were John McCain, who received $546,000, Senate Minority Leader Mitch McConnell, who received $425,000, and Max Baucus, head of the Finance Committee, who received $413,000. Senator Baucus, who did not have significant opposition in his last election and won by a landslide, has endorsed an insurance industry proposal that would force any American who does not have health insurance to buy it.

Even the doctors who are aware of the importance of public health measures often don't speak up. This is foolish, because many policy makers are open to new ideas. I was a participant in the Senate committee hearings on health care in February 2009, along with Dean Ornish, M.D., Mehmet Oz, M.D., and Mark Hyman, M.D.; we were given a very warm reception. My testimony covered many of the same issues that I am presenting in this book, and I'm optimistic that some of my positions will become part of American health care reform.

But significant change will depend on physicians, nurses, pharmacists, and all health professionals actively working to educate their communities, promoting health in schools and workplaces, and becoming involved in the politics of health care. This kind of work will impact millions and should be part of the job descriptions of those who care for our health.

TRAINING THE DOCTOR
OF THE FUTURE

At the Arizona Center for Integrative Medicine we are training a new generation of doctors (as well as medical students, medical residents, and nurse practitioners) to bring integrative medicine to America and the world. We currently offer a comprehensive Fellowship in Integrative Medicine, a one-thousand-hour curriculum taught mostly online, with three residential weeks in Tucson. We have also developed Integrative Medicine in Residency, a two-hundred-hour curriculum that is currently a required, accredited part of eight residency programs around the country. Our long-range goal is to make this a required, accredited part of all residency training in all medical specialties.

We teach the subjects omitted from the conventional curriculum, including complexity, patient individuality, and, especially, the innate healing capacity of the human organism. Our Fellows are encouraged to look beyond symptoms to root causes and to analyze the influence of lifestyle choices on health. And they become familiar with ways of treating illness other than giving drugs.

A recent *New York Times* article described a Harvard Medical School professor who promoted the benefits of cholesterol-lowering drugs and belittled students' concerns about side effects. One student investigated the professor online and found that he was a paid consultant for ten drug companies, including five makers of cholesterol-lowering medications. The student said, "I felt really violated," and joined a group of more than two hundred Harvard students and faculty members who are trying to curtail this corrupting influence. In 2008 Harvard accepted almost $12 million from drug companies, even though the industry has in recent years paid billions of dollars in fines for malfeasance and has been the target of criminal investigations.

The Arizona Center for Integrative Medicine is free of this kind of influence. Our Fellows learn about botanical medicine, mind/body interventions, nutrition, psychology, lifestyle medicine, and other safe, effective methods of triggering the body's ability to heal.

In order to enable these doctors of the future to change patients' behavior for the better, we teach motivational interviewing, a patient-centered communication style that reveals what best motivates individuals. Using this technique, you might ask patients who are smokers what they like about smoking and then ask what they don't like. From there you can elicit why they might want to quit and how they think they can do it. You get them to articulate their values and motives in their own words. Maybe their main motivation is to avoid wrinkles or bad breath rather than fear of lung cancer. Once you get to know how your patients think and what their hopes and fears are, you can help them change.

We also teach "The Healer's Art," a course developed by Rachel Remen, M.D., of the University of California at San Francisco, and now offered at more than fifty medical schools. It covers compassion, intuition, and interactive skills. The four primary sessions of the course are Discovering and Nurturing Your Wholeness; Sharing Grief and Honoring Loss; Beyond Analysis: Allowing Awe in Medicine; and The Care of the Soul. Although it is an elective course (not required), it has become very popular.

Finally, we try to instill in our graduates a sense of the importance of leadership, especially as calls mount for health-care reform. I hope that our active alumni association will evolve into a political action group to effect the transformation of medicine that must be a central part of that reform. One of my life's missions is to see that every doctor who graduates from every medical school receives this kind of comprehensive, healing-oriented, patient-centered medical training.

CHAPTER 6
MEDICINE OF
THE FUTURE

THE BEGINNING OF THE FUTURE

The medicine of the future has already arrived and is available to those who seek it. Throughout America doctors of integrative medicine are practicing in the prevention-oriented, more natural, and cost-effective style that must become standard. Although disease management and high-tech interventions still dominate mainstream practice, integrative medicine has been a growing theme in health care for the past decade.

In 1994 I founded the Program in Integrative Medicine at the University of Arizona Health Sciences Center in Tucson. Although I had but one assistant and a tiny office in a trailer behind the University Medical Center, I had the support of the dean of the College of Medicine, Dr. James Dalen, the first academic leader I met who recognized the need for transformation. He and I agreed that it was essential not only for the welfare of both doctors and patients but also for the creation of a radically different system of health care.

Our program struggled in its early years and met much resistance. To say that the University Medical Center was not hospitable would be an understatement. When we opened an outpatient clinic within the Department of Medicine, we insisted on redesigning several examination rooms to make them more welcoming and let patients know they would have a different kind of medical encounter. We replaced the cold-white fluorescent lighting with soft, incandescent floor and table lamps; installed comfortably padded massage tables in place of the standard metal examination tables; put art on the walls and fresh flowers and plants on desks. The powers that be objected to all these changes. They said that people would trip over the cords of the lamps, increasing liability; that the flowers and plants would cause allergic reactions; and that "regular" doctors wouldn't be able to examine patients on our beautiful massage tables. We let them take away our aroma-therapy diffusers as safety hazards but successfully fought to keep everything else. Over the next few years many patients told us how relaxed they felt discussing their problems with our integrative medicine Fellows in these settings. Eventually even a few of the regular doctors admitted that they preferred to see patients in our rooms.

Jim Dalen took a lot of heat for allowing our program to exist in his institution. A number of his colleagues and prominent medical academics around the country accused him of admitting superstition and New Age nonsense into the halls of science, but he never wavered in his support. Time was on our side. More and more patients wanted integrative medicine, and as the health-care crisis developed, more and more doctors came to us to learn about it and correct the glaring deficiencies in their education and training.

In 2008 the program became the Arizona Center for Integrative Medicine, a center of excellence at the university with an annual budget of $4.5 million, an endowment, a large faculty and staff, and worldwide recognition as the leader in training physicians and allied health professionals to practice medicine more effectively. The Center has graduated more than five hundred physicians, from residents to senior academicians, family doctors and internists, cardiac surgeons and oncologists.

Back in 1994 the term "integrative medicine" was not in common use; few people understood it. As I used it more frequently, my medical colleagues gradually adopted it. I thought the term best described the transformative style of medicine that I knew to be central to health care of the future, and it was free of the negative associations many doctors had to such words as "holistic," "alternative," and "complementary."

"Holistic medicine," popular in the 1970s, suggests treating patients as more than physical bodies — an important concept. But the term has a distinctly New Age ring; moreover, practitioners of holistic medicine often reject conventional treatments and are antagonistic toward those who use them. I consider "whole-person medicine" to be a central principle of integrative medicine (IM), but I avoid the word "holistic." "Alternative medicine" has had a much longer life. Although integrative medicine frequently makes use of alternative therapies in place of pharmaceutical drugs, it never hesitates to rely on conventional methods when those are indicated. We are not trying to replace conventional medicine with something else; rather, we are trying to make it more effective and more cost-effective by broadening its perspective and options for treatment. "Complementary medicine" is another inaccurate description of our practice, because it suggests that we mostly use adjuncts to conventional treatments, add-ons that are secondary and less important. Today, "complementary and alternative" medicine (CAM) is in vogue. We have a National Center for CAM (NCCAM) at NIH. I hope it will soon be renamed the National Center for Integrative Medicine.

Whenever I speak to audiences throughout this country and abroad, I must patiently explain that integrative medicine is not synonymous with CAM. IM will use all appropriate therapies in treating disease, whether conventional or unconventional, as long as they do no harm and are supported by reasonable evidence for efficacy, but it has much broader goals than simply bringing complementary and alternative therapies into mainstream practice. In particular, it aims to do the following:

1. Restore the focus of medical teaching, research, and practice on health and healing;
2. Develop "whole person" medicine, in which the mental, emotional, and spiritual dimensions of human beings are included in diagnosis and

treatment, along with the physical body;

3. Take all aspects of lifestyle into account in assessing health and disease;
4. Protect and emphasize the practitioner/patient relationship as central to the healing process;
5. Emphasize disease prevention and health promotion.

These five goals must characterize American health care in the future, as it rises above the inadequacy of technology-based disease management. As I have said, the ascendancy of technology in the last century inadvertently distorted medical philosophy and practice. Integrative medicine seeks to correct this distortion and reconnect medicine with its roots. That is what attracted Jim Dalen and, later, other academic leaders to it and what now brings so many health-care professionals to our Center for retraining. Our curriculum includes modules on the nature of health and healing, the philosophy and art of medicine, nutrition and health, lifestyle medicine, mind/body interactions, spirituality and health, and botanical medicine — all developed by outstanding medical experts. We also teach our Fellows about alternative therapies and the strengths and weaknesses of traditional systems, such as Chinese medicine and Ayurveda.

The inclusion of alternative therapies in IM is important, because some of them have great potential to lower the cost of health care as well as improve outcomes. I must defend this component of IM; it is the one that attracts the most attention and the harshest criticism.

ACCEPTING THE UNFAMILIAR

Long before I started the original program in integrative medicine, I had investigated other forms of healing around the world: in North America, South America, Africa, India, and East Asia. In these explorations I came across many noteworthy practitioners and treatments that were far afield from the ones I learned at Harvard. Some of the ideas and practices I encountered struck me as nonsensical. Some were clearly in conflict with my scientific understanding. Others seemed strange but worth considering. A few were so sensible and so useful that I wanted to learn more about them and include them in my own practice. I will give a few examples of the best.

Manual Medicine

In the mid-1970s I spent time with an elderly osteopathic physician in Tucson, Robert Fulford, whose particular expertise was in cranial therapy, a gentle, hands-on technique intended to normalize circulatory and respiratory mechanics affecting brain and spinal cord function, a concept undreamt of in conventional medicine. By using this ultra-low-tech, inexpensive method, Dr. Fulford was stunningly effective as a clinician. I watched him cure long-standing chronic conditions, often with one or two sessions of manipulation. For example, he regularly ended recurrent cycles of ear infections (otitis media) in infants and children, a stark contrast to the results of standard treatment — cycles of antibiotics and decongestant drugs, and, sometimes, surgical insertion of tubes in the eardrums.

This experience convinced me that in the hands of a skilled practitioner, manual medicine can be safer and more effective than conventional (usually drug) treatment for common conditions. I made it part of the IM curriculum and continue to work on making it better known and more widely used. (Another accomplished osteopathic physician, Harmon Myers, has been a member of the clinical faculty of our Center since its early days.)

Manual medicine also encompasses chiropractic and the many forms of massage therapy that can be of significant value for muscle pain, stress reduction, and joint dysfunction. An estimated 36 percent of Americans receive a professional massage each year, a majority of them on advice from their doctors. Massage is an important element of sports medicine and can also be beneficial as an adjunctive therapy for people undergoing treatment for serious illnesses, cancer included. I have found specialized forms, such as the Feldenkrais Method, to be remarkably beneficial for rehabilitation from injury and stroke, and often they are more time- and cost-effective than conventional physical therapy.

Traditional and Modern Chinese Medicine

I have seen many successful applications of traditional Chinese medicine, a complex system that includes unique diagnostic methods, massage, dietary and lifestyle adjustment, acupuncture, and herbal therapy. I am even more impressed by the power of modern Chinese medicine, recently developed in China by doctors trained in Western medicine who are matching traditional treatments to conventional pathology. Instead of treating "chi stagnation" in the liver, for example, they are using Chinese herbal formulas to reduce chronic inflammation in that organ and are getting good results that can be studied using Western methods. I have referred patients with serious chronic diseases — including Lyme disease, chronic hepatitis B and C, and autoimmunity — to a colleague in New York, Qingcai Zhang, M.D., who practices in this way. These were patients who had failed to respond to conventional treatment. Most have done well; many have fully regained health with his cheaper, safer, more natural approach.

Dr. Zhang once said to me, "If you could summarize Chinese medical philosophy in one sentence, it would be 'To dispel evil and support the good.'" Western medicine puts all its efforts into "dispelling evil" by fighting germs with antibiotics, giving drugs to lower cholesterol, and destroying malignant tumors by various drastic interventions. It does next to nothing about "supporting the good," meaning the body's natural defenses, its healing system. In my view *both* approaches are necessary. That is what I teach students of integrative medicine. In China today most cancer patients, at least those in cities, receive this kind of comprehensive care. In addition to surgery, radiotherapy, and chemotherapy, they get Chinese treatments, especially sophisticated herbal therapy intended to reduce toxicity and increase the efficacy of radiation and chemotherapy, as well as boost immune defenses against cancer and enhance general health and quality of life. In America very few people with cancer are so fortunate; the demand for integrative cancer care is enormous, but we have only a handful of integrative oncologists in the whole country.

As an isolated therapy, acupuncture can produce dramatic improvement in cases of acute sinusitis, knee effusions, and allergic rhinitis (hay fever). In some people it induces sufficient anesthesia for dental procedures. Scalp acupuncture, a specialized technique mostly practiced in China, is better at speeding recovery from stroke and improving overall function in children with cerebral palsy than any methods of Western medicine.

Botanical Medicine

My long experience with botanical medicine has made me a strong proponent of natural products to treat disease. I find them to be much safer and often more effective than pharmaceutical drugs. Medicinal plants owe their effects to complex mixtures of biologically active compounds. Most pharmaceutical products are single molecules that are highly purified. Western pharmacologists believe that the properties of medicinal plants can be reduced to single "active principles," compounds better delivered to the body in pure form. While it is true that concentrated, purified active principles act rapidly and dramatically, I disagree that they are better, particularly in noncrisis situations. Concentrating pharmacological power also means concentrating toxicity. For example, digitalis (foxglove leaf) is a less powerful heart stimulant than its purified derivative, digoxin, but it is also less dangerous. Crude opium is a less powerful painkiller than morphine or heroin; it is also less addictive. America's current astronomical number of adverse drug reactions — now a leading cause of death in hospitalized patients — is a direct consequence of our enthusiasm for isolated and purified chemical drugs and the medical profession's ignorance of and disdain for diluted complex natural therapeutic agents.

That disdain is rooted in the tendency to ignore the complexity of nature that I mentioned earlier. The arrays of biologically active compounds in plants show ordered patterns in their complexity. One compound is often present in the greatest amount and accounts for most of the effects of a given plant. The many secondary compounds often resemble the dominant one in their chemical structure so that nature's compositions take the form of molecular themes and variations. It is significant that the variant molecules often include both "agonists" and "antagonists" — that is, compounds with opposed pharmacological effects. This accounts for one of the major differences I have observed between medicinal plants and their isolated active principles. The latter cause predictable one-way changes in our physiology; the former have unpredictable and sometimes paradoxical effects that conventional medicine cannot explain. A Chinese herb that can both lower high blood pressure and raise low blood pressure is a baffling puzzle for Western pharmacologists.

The fact is that whole complex natural remedies often have ambivalent effects. They deliver compounds to the body that can both "pull" and "push" our physiology in opposite directions. Which effect will win out, the push or the pull?

One cannot answer that question without using a new model that embraces the complexity of both plants and human beings. The effect that predominates when a patient swallows a remedy made from a whole plant *depends on the state of the patient at the time.* We know that drugs work by binding to specialized receptors on cells or within cells. It is the drug-receptor combination that causes subsequent effects, not the drug alone. Whether the end result of using a complex natural remedy is a push or a pull is a matter of which receptors are available for binding, and that reflects the state of the organism at the time.

I hope I can convey here my excitement at the possibility of a new kind of pharmacotherapeutics. The pharmaceutical drugs that are now the mainstay of conventional medical treatment are very concentrated, powerful, and fast-acting. They give the human organism a strong prod in one direction, allowing it no choice in the matter. There is a place for such treatment, particularly in managing critical conditions when there is no time to waste in restoring the balance of vital functions. In such cases the high risk of toxicity is acceptable. But we are using drugs of this sort for almost every condition, and in most cases the risks (and expense) are not justified.

Complex natural mixtures of pharmacologically active compounds may produce less dramatic, less rapid effects, but they allow the body a choice in how to respond. It gets to participate in the treatment, selecting the actions it needs by making appropriate receptors available. Instead of the outcome being determined solely by the drug, the patient's body can take part in the process to meet its own individualized needs.

I see a secure place for natural products in the medicine of the future, but not necessarily in the form of roots and barks, teas and tonics. We must have access to standardized extracts of medicinal plants that make their actions more predictable and more effective. These must be free of toxic and unwanted constituents and be in forms that doctors are familiar with, such as tablets, capsules, and even injectables, all produced using the same good manufacturing practices in place for pharmaceutical products. I am confident that as doctors and pharmacists learn to use natural therapeutic agents, medical outcomes will improve, adverse reactions will drop sharply, and health-care costs will drop.

Mind/Body Medicine

Over the years I have studied and practiced many forms of mind/body medicine, another core subject of the IM curriculum and one we must stop thinking of as alternative or merely complementary to "real" medicine. It is a well-researched field and has an impressive evidence base built over the past forty years. I therefore find it frustrating that many medical scientists and practitioners still do not see the significance of mind/body interactions and do not make use of therapeutic interventions based on them. The reason is that Western medicine operates from a materialistic paradigm in which the only reality is physical. In this way of thinking, changes in physical systems must have physical causes. Mind/body medicine concerns the nonphysical causation of changes in the body. It is a provocative challenge to conventional assumptions and therefore not welcomed into our medical academies and health-care institutions. Its proponents are often ignored and sometimes ridiculed.

What a shame! Mind/body therapies such as hypnosis, guided imagery, and biofeedback are effective, time efficient, inexpensive, and even enjoyable for both therapists and clients. Their potential to cause harm is very low, particularly compared to that of pharmaceutical drugs. They are useful both as primary treatments and as adjunctive therapies that can reduce side effects and increase the efficacy of other interventions. Over the years I have referred many patients to practitioners of mind/body therapies and have seen many of them improve dramatically or recover completely from chronic pain, allergies, autoimmunity, chronic skin diseases, gastrointestinal disorders, and more. I frequently include these referrals in my treatment plans.

These successes point up a serious defect in the reigning medical paradigm, a defect made much more glaring by recent research that uses new imaging technology to observe living brains. Positron emission tomography (PET) and functional magnetic resonance imaging (f-MRI) scans now allow us to witness brain activity in specific regions and correlate it with mental states and experiences. One pioneer of this research, Richard Davidson, Ph.D., who directs an imaging laboratory at the University of Wisconsin, Madison, has studied Tibetan monks who are adepts at meditation. He has demonstrated consistent differences in their brain function from that of people untrained in meditation, such as the presence of powerful gamma waves — brain waves indicating intensely focused thought — as well as unusual activity of the left prefrontal cortex, which is associated with positive emotions. Other investigators have been able to link placebo responses with activity of a specific brain region. Suddenly, states of consciousness and experiences that materialistic science has been able to dismiss as mystical or unreal can be correlated with real events in the brain. This is a revolutionary development in neuroscience and a strong challenge to the scientific and medical predilection to ignore or discount the influence of mind on body. It certainly points up the foolishness of relegating mind/body therapies to the realm of CAM and refusing to explore their potential to improve medicine and lower the cost of health care.

One common form of mind/body medicine — stress management — has been repeatedly shown to improve physical function and enhance healing. It is estimated that as many as 70 percent of all visits to family doctors are for stress-related disorders, but patients often don't realize the impact of their stressors. Stress can be relieved by a wide variety of methods, including psychotherapy, exercise, reduction in caffeine intake, lifestyle changes, better sleep habits, meditation, and even humor and laughter. My own favorite stress-neutralizing technique is breath work, which is a component of yoga. Breathing bridges the mind/body interface. Regulating it not only promotes relaxation but can also balance the activity of the autonomic (involuntary) nervous system, improving digestion, circulation, and other vital functions. I teach all patients simple breathing exercises. By practicing them, many have been able to wean themselves off drugs they depended on to keep various conditions in check.

The insistence in integrative medicine that patients be treated as whole persons — bodies, minds, spirits, and community members — is intended to correct a fundamental failing of conventional medicine. Even if our IM graduates do not apply mind/body interventions themselves, they know when those interventions are appropriate, for which patients they are most suited, and how to refer to competent therapists. They are also able to discuss with colleagues the scientific evidence supporting these interventions. As the number of health professionals trained in IM grows, I expect to see mind/body medicine move from the fringes to the mainstream — from the CAM of today to the conventional medicine of to-morrow.

Nutritional Medicine

The power of dietary adjustment to help the body heal has been vastly underestimated within our disease management system, and until relatively recently, nutrition was not even considered a significant factor in disease causation and prevention. For example, experts argued for many years that diet had little influence on one's risk for cancer. Now it is widely accepted that high-fat diets raise the risk of breast, prostate, and other hormonally driven tumors, that diets low in fiber raise the risk of colorectal cancer, and that many specific foods and nutrients have cancer-protective effects.

Although the medical profession now generally regards diet as an important factor in disease prevention, few practitioners recommend dietary change as a primary therapeutic strategy. Integrative medicine doctors do that all the time. For example, they know that type-2 diabetes can be prevented by attending to good nutrition and can also be controlled in many patients by dietary adjustment, especially in combination with adequate physical activity. The conditions that respond to dietary interventions range from autistic disorders to depression, allergies and autoimmunity to chronic sinusitis, recurrent bladder infections to migraines.

Obesity, which contributes to hypertension, heart disease, stroke, cancer (particularly of the breast, uterus, colon, kidney, and esophagus), type-2 diabetes, and joint dysfunction, is a major American problem. The diseases associated with it account for a large percentage of our health-care expenditures, an estimated yearly total of $117 billion. The cause of epidemic obesity in America is our eating habits, which have changed greatly in my lifetime. A robust enterprise of nutritional medicine could help us correct them.

Many of the costly chronic degenerative illnesses, particular those that affect people over sixty (cardiovascular disease, cancer, Alzheimer's) are rooted in inappropriate inflammation. Most people in our country eat pro-inflammatory diets that are full of harmful fats and refined carbohydrates that raise blood sugar too quickly. They do not get enough good fats (like omega-3's from oily fish that reduce inflammation) or protective nutrients from fruits and vegetables. I have been promoting an anti-inflammatory diet for several years. It is not hard to follow because it is based on the Mediterranean diet and includes many enjoyable foods, from olive oil and pasta to dark chocolate (and red wine for those who want it).

Nutritional medicine is a cornerstone of IM. In our new health-care system, doctors must be able to advise patients how to eat well to achieve and maintain optimum wellness and how to adjust eating patterns to modify conditions that affect health.

Dietary Supplementation

Supplementation with vitamins, minerals, essential fatty acids, and other natural products can promote health, prevent disease, and contribute to successful treatment. Ideally, all nutrients should be obtained from the diet. Supplements are not substitutes for whole foods. Multivitamin products are, at best, only partial representations of the complex arrays of micronutrients in foods. Nonetheless, dietary supplements, including vitamins and minerals, can be useful as insurance against gaps in the diet. It is most important to get the correct amounts and forms of micronutrients from supplements. For example, nature produces vitamin E as a complex of eight molecules, but most multivitamins contain only one of those, alpha-tocopherol. (And that lone component is also what reductionistically-minded researchers have studied, which may account in part for their failure to document the health benefits of taking vitamin E.)

Most people are confused about dietary supplements, particularly with so much contradictory information, misinformation, and, I'm sorry to say, disinformation circulating about them. People need guidance here, guidance that should come from physicians and pharmacists, not from health food store clerks and commercial Web sites. Today's professional training does not prepare doctors and pharmacists to do that. The Arizona Center for Integrative Medicine is teaching physicians and nurse-practitioners what they need to know about the benefits, risks, and appropriate uses of dietary supplements; soon it will be teaching pharmacists as well.

Physical Activity

The evidence base for the powerful role of physical activity in promoting and maintaining health, preventing disease, and speeding healing is nothing short of massive. If you want to live a long and healthy life, you must be physically active and remain physically active. One of the most constant findings about healthy old people is that they have maintained physical activity throughout life. That does not mean they ran marathons, went to aerobics classes, and had personal trainers. They might simply have walked every day, done housework, or gardened, but they did so energetically and regularly. As recently as the early 1900s, most people in America were physically active for at least five hours every day, working on farms or in factories, walking a great deal, and doing chores at home. At that time about 40 percent of all people lived on farms, and 80 percent of all farm work was done with human labor. This degree of activity was the norm throughout human history, until the last several decades.

Exercise doesn't just burn calories and protect us from the consequences of overeating. It has innumerable beneficial effects on the body and mind. It improves cardiac function and the elasticity of arteries, allowing more blood flow to all tissues and organs. It increases perspiration and the exchange of oxygen and carbon dioxide, both of which help eliminate the waste products of metabolism. It boosts the brain's production of endorphins (our natural painkillers and antidepressants) by almost 500 percent and raises levels of the neurotransmitter dopamine, another mood elevator. It helps prevent age-related dementia. It makes cells more sensitive to insulin, stabilizing blood sugar and lowering risks of obesity and type-2 diabetes.

Studies indicate that regular aerobic exercise substantially decreases the risk of breast cancer and colon cancer. It also helps alleviate chronic pain.

Strength training builds and maintains muscle and bone. Good muscle mass equates with efficient metabolism and calorie burning. Good bone density offers protection against osteoporosis and the associated risk of hip fracture in the elderly (a common cause of premature disability and death).

Flexibility and balance training are vital for protecting joints so that they will allow the body to be physically active throughout life. Balance training is of special importance for older people who are at greater risk for fractures from falls. In fact, a recent study showed that it was more effective than bone-building drugs at preventing fractures.

For all these reasons, our integrative medicine curriculum has a strong focus on physical activity as a key component of health promotion and as a way of treating disease.

All the therapies I have discussed are currently relegated to the world of CAM and are marginal to mainstream medicine. Integrating them with the best of conventional practices is one of the major goals of IM in order to greatly improve American health care and make it much more affordable.

THE EARLY DAYS OF THE NEW MEDICINE

Soon after I returned from my travels and settled in the desert outside of Tucson, Arizona, in the mid-1970s, I began to see patients at my home. I first described what I did as "natural and preventive medicine." Later I came to call it integrative medicine, because I wanted people to know that I combined the conventional medicine I had learned at Harvard with ideas and practices from other systems and traditions. I explained that IM neither rejects conventional medicine nor embraces alternative therapies uncritically. In fact, I have always taught that the worst mistake an IM practitioner can make is to miss the diagnosis of a condition that should go straight to standard care. In other words: Send a patient with possible acute appendicitis to an emergency room, not to a hypnotherapist.

Even in those early days it was obvious to me that there was great demand for the service I offered. Those who came to me were frustrated with their health care. They had not been helped or had been harmed by conventional medicine and wanted to take greater responsibility for their own well-being. They were overjoyed to be able to sit with a medical doctor who was open-minded about treatments other than drugs and surgery; who took the time to listen to their stories; who gave advice about diet and products in health food stores and alternative therapies; and who could help them figure out their best options for treatment. I was delighted that some of the people who sought me out were in good health and simply wanted to know more about how to maintain it.

Most of the patients I saw had been through the medical mill many times. They brought extensive medical records and results of diagnostic workups, so I rarely had to worry about missing problems that required standard treatment. If I thought some possibility had been overlooked, I would send the patient to an internist or specialist whom I knew and trusted. Most of my consultations lasted an hour. At the end of that time I would give my impressions along with a treatment plan that addressed not only the presenting problem but other issues that caught my attention. My treatment plans included dietary recommendations (about both foods and supplements), other lifestyle advice (about exercise, for example, and use of alcohol and caffeine), information about botanical remedies, instructions for breath work and other relaxation methods, and suggested reading. I also made referrals to other practitioners, most frequently mind/body therapists (for hypnotherapy or guided imagery), osteopathic physicians (for manipulation), practitioners of traditional Chinese medicine, psychotherapists, and teachers of yoga and meditation.

Patients came to see me from far and wide, many for a one-time consultation to get direction on the path to better health. I asked all of them to report on their progress two months after the visit, or sooner if they had more questions or new problems. The follow-up communications I received reinforced my conviction that the integrative approach worked well for many people and many health conditions. It was especially gratifying to learn of recoveries from chronic illnesses that had not responded to standard treatment.

I am quick to admit that much of my clinical success had to do with the kinds of patients I saw. I do not mean that they had trivial problems. Quite the opposite: Many presented with very difficult multisystem diseases that would be challenging for any practitioner and any system of medicine. Some came to see me as a last resort, with advanced life-threatening conditions. But they were all self-selected patients who were highly motivated to make changes in their lives. They sought good information, answers to questions, and sound advice. Compliance was not an issue; they were eager to take greater control of their lives and more than willing to implement the suggestions I gave them.

One of the greatest rewards of practicing IM is that you attract such motivated patients. Motivated patients are a pleasure to work with. It is easy to mobilize their innate healing potential, which increases the probability that simple treatments and targeted lifestyle changes will produce the desired results. The frustration of many doctors today is that they have to work in impersonal settings with patients who think of their bodies as appliances brought into the shop for repair. That attitude, especially with insufficient time to form a productive therapeutic relationship, reduces the likelihood of clinical success and true healing.

INTEGRATIVE MEDICINE: OBSTACLES AND OPPORTUNITIES

Although individual physicians came to me to learn about the kind of medicine I practiced, for a long time it was more popular with the public than with most of my colleagues. Academic health centers did not show any receptivity to IM until the mid-1990s. All that has changed. Almost a third of the nation's medical schools are now members of the Consortium of Academic Health Centers for Integrative Medicine (www.imconsortium.org). Why did things change? The answer is simple: economics. As long as it was business as usual in American health care, no amount of ideological argument about the limitations of conventional medicine moved anything. Never mind that Americans were spending more on CAM practitioners than on visits to primary care physicians or that sales of dietary supplements and herbal remedies climbed into the billions. Only the worsening economic squeeze opened institutional medicine to change.

As other IM programs appeared and medical students signed up for elective courses in CAM, opposition soon developed. IM is a strong and growing movement in the United States today, and if it were not so strong, it would not be the target of such vocal criticism. Most of that criticism comes from defenders of scientific orthodoxy who accuse me and other leaders of the movement of promoting unscientific or even antiscientific ideas and practices. Their negativity is one obstacle to correcting the glaring disparities of insurance reimbursement that impede the growth of IM and ensure that health-care costs will continue to resist all efforts to contain them.

The fact is that American medicine is reimbursement driven, not evidence driven. Doctors, hospitals, and clinics provide only those treatments and services that insurers pay for. Lack of reimbursement is the main challenge confronting doctors who want to practice IM. Our dysfunctional health-care system happily pays for costly and often ineffective procedures and drugs but not for preventive counseling or most unconventional therapies, even those that are safe, effective, and cheap. The most inelastic factor in managed care is the practitioner's time. With the corporatization of American health care, the time that doctors are allotted to spend with patients has been sharply curtailed, and that could get worse. In many clinics in Japan today "two-minute doctors" see thirty patients an hour! It is inconceivable to me that good medical care can be delivered in such straitened circumstances. I have long argued that investing in an initial visit of an hour or more will lead to net savings down the road, including less need for practitioners' time, fewer future visits, and less use of expensive procedures and medications. Of course, that proposition needs to be proved by assessing outcomes and costs of integrative versus standard care and presenting the data to those who pay for health care.

An initial integrative medical assessment commonly requires a sixty- to ninety-minute visit in order for the practitioner to take a comprehensive history. Most doctors who try to practice that way have great difficulty getting reimbursed for their time. Some juggle standardized billing codes to get paid more; others try to submit alternative billing codes that place greater value on lifestyle counseling. Most end up asking patients to pay for integrative services out-of-pocket or offering to help them seek reimbursement from insurers.

175

What saddens me most about this situation is that it makes integrative medicine available to the affluent and denies it to those without means. This major roadblock is obstructing the transformation of medicine and must be removed.

As consumer spending on CAM has increased, some insurers have begun to offer plans that cover acupuncture, manual medicine, stress reduction training, and other alternative therapies. In general, however, patients who venture outside of conventional medicine have no hope of being reimbursed for treatment, and none of the big health insurance companies have yet embraced integrative medicine in its totality. They do not yet realize how much money it can save them.

I hope that the private sector in our country can be of help here. Large American corporations are so hobbled by rising health-care costs that they are willing to try any measures to contain them. Unlike the NIH and the rest of the medical research community, corporate health directors have no preconceptions about outcomes studies involving novel therapies and complex interventions. They just want to know what works and how they can maintain the health of their employees without spending more and more. Corporations could take the lead in organizing the outcomes studies we so desperately need, perhaps in creative partnerships with government.

One of the initiatives of the Arizona Center is the Corporate Health Improvement Program (CHIP), under the direction of Dr. Kenneth R. Pelletier. It is a research and development program of the University of Arizona College of Medicine in collaboration with selected Fortune 500 companies and government agencies. (Among the members are Corning, Dow, Ford, IBM, NASA, Prudential, and the Republic of Singapore.) CHIP's current focus is on integrative medicine's clinical effectiveness and cost-effectiveness to corporate America. Dr. Pelletier is optimistic about the program, because he feels that corporations are "the largest segment of our society with a vested interest in health." It goes without saying that most of the health-care industry has a vested interest in disease management.

Some members of CHIP have ongoing research projects, such as a randomized clinical trial at Ford Motor Company on an integrative medicine intervention for back pain. This is not quite the kind of outcomes study we need most, but the interest of large corporations in innovative approaches to health care gives me hope.

I asked Dr. Pelletier about the prospects for doing broader kinds of research. He told me that although determining efficacy and cost outcomes for IM in the workplace has been CHIP's main thrust in recent years, progress has been slow. "Interest in this and receptivity to integrative medicine are not the problem. Funding is," he told me. "Getting money for outcomes studies is tough even in conventional medicine. NIH and CDC are not very helpful, and few private foundations and donors are interested. We have secured a few IM grants from CHIP members." He further commented that within large corporations there is little common language between chief financial officers and chief medical officers.

If lack of funding is the immediate reason for the lack of outcomes studies comparing the clinical effectiveness and cost-effectiveness of integrative versus conventional medicine, then we must take the following actions:

- Convince the CFOs of American corporations of the vital importance of getting this information. It could provide immediate help in reducing their health-care spending.

- Determine the health conditions that now cost corporations the most. For those in which IM shows promise, set up smaller, less expensive pilot studies that can provide data to support larger definitive studies.
- Do the same for the population at large. The health insurance industry knows very well what diseases and conditions cost the most to manage: heart disease, cancer, trauma, mental disorders, diabetes, hypertension, and back problems. The industry should be a partner in conducting pilot outcomes trials to get preliminary data on more cost-effective ways of managing these disorders.
- Direct the U.S. Department of Health and Human Services (HHS) to allocate funds for this research. The Agency for Healthcare Research and Quality (AHRQ) would be the logical division to coordinate it, but it has thus far shown no interest. NIH should participate. It must broaden its mission to include clinical outcomes studies, support the development of new research methodology to study complex, individualized treatments, and

fund the training of investigators to use it.

- Develop collaborations among government agencies, corporations, and foundations interested in health care to make the necessary outcomes studies happen. Under Dr. Julie Gerberding, the CDC awarded health protection research initiative grants that, in part, support research "to develop effective health promotion and prevention programs at the workplace." This initiative should be strengthened and better focused.
- If, as my colleagues and I believe, the results show that IM produces outcomes as good or better and at less expense than those of conventional treatment, then the same collaborations should use their influence to change policies of reimbursement in health care.

Together, all of these constitute a prerequisite for transforming medicine, with the intent of making it less dependent on costly technology-based interventions for the management of common health conditions.

Integrative medicine has been the focus of my professional life for the past three decades. As you can see, I am passionate about its potential to improve our health and heal our ailing health-care system. There are other encouraging trends in American medicine. Terms like "patient-centered medicine" and "spirituality and medicine" are now in common use on campuses of academic health centers. Many thoughtful physicians are working to increase awareness of cultural factors affecting health and outcomes of medical encounters. (For example, Hmong patients coming to a clinic in Minneapolis may have very different perceptions of symptoms and procedures from those of the American doctors seeing them.) And many providers are trying to bring better health care to impoverished communities.

All of this helps, but I believe integrative medicine, with its comprehensive philosophy and rational practices, is the specific corrective needed to get American medicine back on track. IM doctors are ideally qualified to practice the kinds of preventive and lifestyle medicine I have described. Along with like-minded nurses, pharmacists, and others, they are best positioned to improve our dismal health outcomes and create a functional, cost-effective health-care system that serves all of our citizens.

A CONSERVATIVE APPROACH

Two years ago I was invited to speak about my work and my thoughts on the future of health care to groups of doctors and a large public audience in Charlotte, North Carolina, where one of the first graduates of the University of Arizona fellowship training, Russ Greenfield, M.D., had established an IM clinical center. From the moment I was picked up in the baggage claim area of the Charlotte airport until I walked onstage to give my evening lecture, I was repeatedly warned to be careful about what I would say. All my self-appointed advisers began with the very same caution: "Charlotte, you know, is a *very* conservative place."

I opened my talk by saying that if Charlotte is a very conservative place, as I had heard so often since my arrival, then it should be very receptive to integrative medicine, which is fundamentally a conservative movement.

- It is *philosophically* conservative in that it aims to restore core values of medicine that were strong in the past, such as reverence for the healing power of nature and the importance of the therapeutic relationship.
- It is *medically* conservative in stressing

prevention and advocating lesser rather than greater intervention — the least invasive, least harmful, least expensive treatments that the circumstances of illness demand. IM practitioners always observe the Hippocratic precept of "First, do no harm," relying on simpler interventions whenever possible and turning to more drastic ones only when the former fail to produce desired outcomes.

- It is *fiscally* conservative in its willingness to look beyond the borders of conventional medicine to identify inexpensive therapies that may be useful and in its insistence that they be compared to standard therapies for clinical effectiveness and cost-effectiveness in well-designed outcomes trials.

I was not run out of town and have even been invited to return to Charlotte to say more.

■ ■ ■ ■

PART III
HOW TO GET THERE

■ ■ ■ ■

CHAPTER 7
THE NEW AMERICAN
HEALTH CARE

American health care can, will, and *must* be transformed into an enterprise that is less expensive and more effective than our current failed system of disease management. A new system, based on integrative medicine and emphasizing disease prevention and health promotion, is our only practical option for restoring the health of millions of Americans and the health of our economy. The present medical style of high-tech disease intervention, which costs America *one-sixth* of all our earnings, is obsolete. It is completely ill-suited to the chronic lifestyle diseases that now disable and kill most Americans. Replacing it with a radically different model of health care will be one of the most important social movements of our young century.

The mark of success of the integrative medicine movement that I have helped develop will allow us to drop the word "integrative." At that point we will simply have *good medicine* that meets the needs of American patients, government, and business. It will be sustainable far into the future. In this section I will tell you how this transformation can occur and paint a picture of what health care of the future can be.

It will not look like today's overpriced, overcomplicated hierarchical system of late-stage intervention in long-term illness. It will not be dictated by the insurance companies, dominated by the pharmaceutical companies, marked by revolving-door corporate employment, or protected by politicians hungry for campaign financing. Today's conventional, high-tech medicine *will* play a role in tomorrow's health care, but I see it more as a specialty, practiced in specialized centers. Recall that appropriate use of conventional methods is a central tenet of IM, with emphasis on "appropriate." Knowing when and when not to use technology-based diagnostic tools and treatments is critical. We currently use them for practically every health problem that comes through the door. *In the future we must use them only for those patients and those conditions where benefit-to-cost ratios are favorable.*

Conventional medicine is most appropriate for the diagnosis and treatment of severe advanced illness and injury, disease involving vital organs, and other critical conditions. Such cases represent only about 20 percent of all the health problems that physicians see. The greatest cost savings we can get in American health care — which will also result in improved outcomes — will come from *limiting* the use of expensive diagnostic and therapeutic methods to those cases for which they are clearly indicated.

THE TWO CRITICAL CHANGES

The most fundamental change in the health care of the future will be the replacement of widespread use of pharmaceutical drugs by more cost-effective treatments that achieve better results. At various points in this book I have expressed my dismay at the unprecedented extent of pharmaceutical drug consumption in our society today. As with other aspects of technology-based medicine, drugs have a secure place in critical care, terminal care, and the management of severe disease. But in my vision for the transformation of medicine, pharmaceuticals play a much smaller role in the treatment of common conditions, because both doctors and patients will be knowledgeable about other less expensive and less dangerous interventions that work.

Many drugs are not only ineffective but have dangers that are frequently played down (and occasionally concealed) by manufacturers. Adverse drug reactions account for a great deal of unnecessary illness and death. These dangers are frequently not recognized by the medical community, partly because of deception by the drug companies. One study of drug brochures given to doctors found that more than 10 percent contained data that were different from the actual data found in studies. The FDA is supposed to protect the public from this kind of harm, but it is understaffed, underfunded, and has a long and worsening history of protecting the interests of the pharmaceutical industry more than those of public health. Congress has thus far been unable or unwilling to stand up to the extraordinarily vigorous pharmaceutical lobby and institute any sort of price controls on prescription drugs — even for the federal Medicare program.

These grave problems, like so many problems with health care, stem from greed, pure and simple. The pharmaceutical industry reaps egregious profits. The markup on prescription drugs is greater than on almost any other category of products. The companies justify this by claiming that they must spend large sums on research and development. In fact, those expenditures are dwarfed by the amounts spent on advertising and promotion. In 2005 the top five U.S. drug companies had total sales of $222 billion. They spent $32 billion of that on R & D but over twice that much — $71 billion — on marketing and promotion.

Despite this, the U.S. government gives rich tax breaks and subsidies to pharmaceutical companies for new drug development — more than any other government does. Nine of the twenty largest drug companies in the world are based in the United States, but drugs are more expensive here than anywhere else, and global drug companies make most of their profits here. American companies don't even make most of their drugs here. Seventy-five to 80 percent of all active ingredients used in American drugs are now imported, primarily from China and India, and approximately 40 percent of all finished dosage forms are manufactured abroad. Because of this the FDA in one recent year was able to inspect only one-third of the 3,250 international facilities that manufacture American drugs and drug ingredients.

Drug manufacturers unduly influence medical practice through the activity of representatives who cajole and bribe doctors and hospitals to use their products. "The influence that the pharmaceutical companies are having on every aspect of medicine . . . is so blatant now you'd have to be deaf, blind, and dumb not to see it," said *Journal of the American Medical Association* editor Dr. Catherine DeAngelis. "We have just allowed them to take over, and it's our fault, the whole medical community."

The second most important aspect of health-care reform must be to halt the exploitation of Americans by the insurance industry. This extraordinarily wealthy industry drives the cost of health care up and its quality down. The health insurance industry is in lockstep with the pharmaceutical industry, and we all end up paying for the collusion. To take on these megacorporations we will need to mobilize our citizens' widespread frustration and anger with the industry's abusive practices and profiteering. The big companies will resist any attempts at regulation as unacceptable government interference with business, and their lobbies are powerfully influential in Washington. (They spent $138 million in 2007 — not, you can be sure, in support of legislation for universal health care.) I believe, however, that the millions of Americans who have been denied coverage and claims, resulting in inability to get needed treatments — as well as financial ruin — can raise their collective voice and overwhelm the influence of the lobbyists. This is the only way we will be able to force Congress to stop protecting the industry. As citizens and voters we must insist that our Congress serve *us* instead of its corporate masters.

We must also leave behind our naive faith in high-tech medical equipment, including the "wonderful" imaging devices that are now so popular. Americans are now exposed to seven times as much cancer-causing radiation as they were in 1980, and twice as much as in 2000 (at a cost of $14 billion), but much of this exposure provides no benefit whatsoever. As I've noted, a great deal of imaging is done more for profit than the protection of patients; it occurs approximately three times more often in the offices of doctors who own their own imaging devices. Screening for early detection of disease, in general, seems on the surface to be a good idea, but it often leads patients to unnecessary further testing or treatment and is sometimes completely unnecessary.

New Ways to Learn

To stop the runaway cost and declining effectiveness of medicine, our new health care must depend on reformed medical education and research. The curriculums of medical schools must include required courses on health, healing, and lifestyle influences on disease. In addition we should insist that medical schools give students instruction in and an opportunity to practice health-promoting habits *themselves.* We should also insist that they evaluate applicants not only on the basis of intelligence and academic achievement but also on their health habits and potential for modeling healthy living. Finally, we must require that all medical residency training include a comprehensive integrative medicine curriculum.

Changes must also occur in the education and training of nurses, pharmacists, and other health professionals; they must attain a basic level of knowledge about nutrition, lifestyle medicine, mind/body interactions, and complementary and alternative therapies. Pharmacists must learn about appropriate uses of botanical remedies, dietary supplements, and other natural therapeutic agents, as well as their possible interactions with prescription and over-the-counter drugs. Pharmacists should be able to advise both doctors and consumers about these products and assess the accuracy of information about them that comes from manufacturers and distributors, Internet sites, and health food store employees.

We also need to wrest control of medical research from the pharmaceutical companies, who now fund a great deal of it and get the results they want from randomized controlled trials. And we need to change *what* we research, especially looking at interventions other than drugs. We must get necessary outcomes and effectiveness studies underway — or at least start preliminary pilot studies — to compare the clinical effectiveness and cost-effectiveness of integrative treatment versus conventional treatment for common conditions that consume most of our health-care dollars. We need outcomes data to convince payers to change their policies of reimbursement, which now skew health care away from prevention and health promotion.

The keys to making these changes are already in our hands. We can start to use them today both to improve our own health and to build a system that works for all of us.

CHAPTER 8
DISEASE PREVENTION: THE SUSTAINABLE SOLUTION

FROM INTERVENTION TO PREVENTION

The word "prevention" derives from two Latin roots that mean "before" and "come." The concept is that by anticipating what may come that can harm us, we can take action to stop it, avert it, or minimize its effects.

There are two requirements for the effective prevention of disease, reflecting the word's two component roots: being able to foresee danger and taking appropriate action to avoid it. In matters of health, prevention would seem to be straightforward. We can prevent some serious infectious diseases by immunizing against them. We can often avoid colds by washing our hands. We can greatly reduce the incidence of lung cancer, emphysema, and other dire conditions by curtailing tobacco addiction. In practice, however, the prevention of disease is far from straightforward.

Even if we can identify proper preventive measures, we may not be able to implement them. Is that why we as a society do such a poor job of prevention? How can we explain why we are stuck in the present costly mode of disease management even though it is obvious that prevention is the better approach, medically and fiscally? The obstacles to progress are complex. Some are created by insurance companies, which are unwilling to pay for prevention; others are created by pharmaceutical companies, which persuade doctors and patients to rely on drugs to maintain health. Our health professionals are not well trained in prevention. Few doctors know how to motivate patients to change behavior and make better lifestyle choices. And most Americans, I'm sorry to say, would rather pop pills than make the effort that prevention requires.

The disproportion between the time, money, and energy spent in coping with established disease — i.e., intervention — versus the time, money, and energy spent on prevention is huge. It is one facet of the crisis that has brought the American health-care system to the point of collapse. We must understand why our efforts at disease prevention are so limited and so feeble, and how we can make them strong and effective.

The chronic diseases that are now epidemic in America are largely preventable. Over the past century, acute infectious illness was replaced as America's major health problem by chronic degenerative disease. This striking change was a strong driver of the rising expense of health care that now overwhelms us. Lifestyle factors figure prominently in the causation of chronic disease: obesity, smoking, lack of physical activity, unmanaged exposure to toxins, etc., and can therefore best be addressed by integrative medicine. The same basic elements of lifestyle medicine that I described in chapter 5 can not only control (and sometimes reverse) chronic diseases but can also help prevent them. Most of the chronic degenerative diseases, including the age-related ones that are responsible for so much disability in our graying population, result from interactions between genes and environmental factors. Many of the latter reflect the ways we choose to live and so are under our control. For example, many cases of cancer in our population are correlated with smoking, obesity, diet, and exposure to toxins.

Consider these facts about our current

chronic disease epidemic:

The Toll of Preventable Disease

- Chronic diseases cause 70 percent of deaths in America and are responsible for three-fourths of health-care spending.
- Half of all American men and one-third of all American women will develop cancer.
- One-fourth of all Americans will have heart disease.
- One in twelve Americans will have asthma.
- One in fourteen Americans will have diabetes.
- One in seven Americans will develop Alzheimer's disease.

These chronic diseases are not inevitable consequences of growing older. When I lecture about healthy aging, I am always asked, "How much of our destiny is genetically determined?" It is probably not possible to give a precise numerical answer, but from my reading of the scientific literature and my discussions with experts, I have concluded that the human body is genetically designed not only to last but to function well all the way into our eighties. While we may need rare inherited traits — what some researchers call "genetic booster rockets" — to maintain health and vigor into our late nineties and beyond, many recent discoveries show that environment and lifestyle factors can modify genetic expression and influence risk for age-related disease.

Genes turn on and off. Most of the ones we have in all our cells are inactive. We have long known that hormones (such as insulin and estrogen) and other biochemical regulators (such as melatonin and prostaglandins) produce their effects by activating specific genes. One exciting area of research — nutrigenomics — has found that certain nutrients can also do this. What a woman eats during pregnancy may influence genetic expression in her baby. What a man with prostate cancer eats may switch cancer-protective genes on or off. One study showed that women who maintain a healthy weight and manage their stress well appear to be less likely than obese or stressed women to have age-related chromosomal changes. Even more provocative is a bit of evidence that emotions alone can have the same effect — that relaxation training can turn off genes responsible for harmful effects of stress and that laughter can turn off some of the genes that control the expression of type-2 diabetes.

Even if we have insufficient data to convince the evidence-based medical community of the power of lifestyle factors to modify gene expression, we can easily observe it in our own experience. Many Americans today are aging in ways different from their parents and grandparents. "Seventy is the new sixty" and "Sixty is the new fifty" are now familiar sayings in our culture, and for many of our seventy- and sixty-year-olds, these slogans are true. What has changed? Not genes, certainly. A population does not undergo significant genetic change in the course of one or two generations. What has changed is how people live. Many aging Americans now have more knowledge about healthy living and greater access to health-promoting products and services (including medical services) than their parents and grandparents had, and this enables them to age more gracefully.

Unfortunately, in contrast to those who are enjoying healthier lives are the much greater number who are leading careless lifestyles and suffering from chronic diseases. The CDC estimates that each year 1.7 million Americans die and 25 million more are disabled by chronic diseases that are caused or exacerbated by lifestyle factors. A recent study reported in the *New England Journal of Medicine* predicted that, due to current lifestyle factors, American life expectancy will decline in the next twenty years, after having increased regularly since the 1850s.

This is why I believe that the lifestyle component of integrative medicine should be the main thrust of tomorrow's preventive health care. It offers the best and most cost-effective possibilities for decreasing the incidence of the diseases that now absorb so many of our health-care dollars. Lifestyle medicine includes public education about the influence of lifestyle choices on disease risks; modeling of healthy living by physicians and other health-care professionals; societal efforts to make better lifestyle choices fashionable and affordable; and personal efforts to live in ways that reduce risks of chronic disease.

OBSTACLES TO PREVENTION

What stands in the way of our doing this today?

- Doctors and patients in our country want quick fixes. Drugs appear to be quick fixes. We need to discard this way of thinking.

- Because there is widespread ignorance about the relative importance of factors under our control that influence risks of disease, we have little or no motivation to change behavior. For example, most women are surprised to learn that excess weight and obesity cause more cases of breast cancer than genes or environmental toxins.

- Many of us are lazy and resistant to changing our ways *or* don't believe we can *or* think it requires us to stop doing everything we enjoy. We would rather have something done *to* us or *for* us. We need to take responsibility for our own well-being and long-term health.

- Doctors and nurses too often exemplify behaviors that need to change rather than inspire patients by modeling healthy living. A doctor who is overweight is unlikely to persuade a patient to lose weight. As Harvard's Walter Willett, M.D., recently noted, "[Doctors] tend to feel inhibited in counseling others when they aren't exactly setting an example." This must end if we are to inspire patients to make positive changes.

- Our hospitals and medical centers are hardly supportive environments in which to teach people to improve their lives. Their architecture, interior design, aesthetics, odors, and isolation from nature are all inimical to health and healing — not to mention the food they serve. (Almost 40 percent of American hospitals have fast-food restaurants on their premises.)
- Some of our government's unenlightened policies make it *harder* for Americans to make better choices in life. Glaring examples are federal subsidies that make unhealthy food cheap, and healthy food expensive. The Department of Agriculture subsidizes the production of corn and soy, with the result that harmful derivatives of those crops (high-fructose corn syrup, refined soy oil) are so cheap that they are ubiquitous in the processed and manufactured foods Americans consume in vast quantities. There are no subsidies for growing fruits and vegetables; the resulting high prices for them explains their relatively low consumption. Other examples of U.S. government policies that directly lead

to worse, not better, health of its citizens are anticonservation rulings, which are too numerous to detail here, that damage the quality of our air, soil, and water, and the lack of funding for public schools that results in the elimination of physical education classes. The government must become the friend of healthy living, not the enemy.

- The big food manufacturers persuade many people, kids especially, to eat the unhealthiest forms of refined and processed foods, such as soft drinks and sugar-laden breakfast cereals. American corporations must be aligned with societal efforts to improve the lifestyles and health of our citizens. And why shouldn't they? The corporate bottom line suffers when the health of the workforce suffers.

- Our priorities of insurance reimbursement are backward. Insurers pay for the use of prescription drugs as a primary means of prevention, but these drugs are often very expensive and minimally effective. Insurers do not pay doctors for lifestyle counseling or reimburse patients for the cost of services, equipment, and products that help them change behavior and live in ways that reduce risks of disease.

This book is a call for radical change. We can remove all these barriers, but only if individuals, government, and the private sector work together toward a common goal. We cannot have the government telling us to eat better while continuing to make unhealthy foods cheaper than healthy ones. Corporate America needs to realize it cannot compete in the global economy if it is saddled with the expenses of managing the high prevalence of chronic illness. And we cannot allow the health insurance and pharmaceutical industries to call the shots in preventive medicine.

I am not going to leave you in despair about the magnitude of these obstacles. I will offer specific recommendations, including actions that you as an individual citizen can take to bring about a more effective enterprise of preventive medicine as well as a new specialty of lifestyle medicine. These will be core components of a better system of health care that will improve our lagging health outcomes without dragging us into bankruptcy.

Assume we've done it. The new system is in place. Your health insurance will now fully pay for appointments with a new kind of doctor, a clinical specialist in preventive medicine. And it will pay preventive doctors enough to make these consultations worth their time, so they won't have to rush through them. What might you expect from the visit?

The more information you can provide in advance about your personal health history, family history, and lifestyle, the better. Medical information will soon be centralized and easily available in electronic form. In addition, progress in genomics and the determination of the entire DNA sequence of organisms will make it possible to identify individual genetic predispositions for disease. For example, if your major inherited risk is coronary artery disease, your preventive medical consultation will focus on all that you can do, starting as early in life as possible, to modify the expression of relevant genes and protect the health of your heart and blood vessels. This will include advice about conventional medical diagnostic testing, monitoring, and treatment, if necessary, as well as lifestyle recommendations. If, instead, Alzheimer's disease appears as your chief inherited risk, you will learn what strategies are available to protect brain health and mental function and reduce the likelihood of your getting it.

Your doctor will not only help you understand this information but will also motivate you to use it by giving you detailed instructions — meal plans, for example — and by modeling healthy living for you. He or she will also refer you to other professionals, such as nutritionists and stress-management trainers, and connect you with groups and services to support your efforts. You will come away from the visit knowing the benefits and risks of medications you take. You will also learn about any dietary supplements that will be useful for you and how to be an informed and careful consumer of health-care products and alternative medical services.

Your preventive care will include setting goals that you and your doctor agree are important and attainable, with follow-up monitoring of your progress. All this will extend throughout your life, making it easier for you to anticipate and adapt to age-related changes. *You* will be the most important decision maker in your lifelong health care, not some insurance company or clinic or even a physician. Insurance companies will make this kind of care affordable, and you will, of course, enroll your children in it in their earliest years.

OPPORTUNITIES FOR PREVENTION

There are a number of lifestyle and behavioral changes that you can make starting today. Dietary modification can dramatically lower disease risks. Start by reducing intake (and eventually eliminating consumption) of refined, processed, and manufactured foods. Increase physical activity; avoid obesity; don't smoke; take appropriate dietary supplements; learn and practice techniques of stress management; and get adequate rest and sleep. Each of these factors is important individually, but in combination their effectiveness is much greater. Lifestyle choices also influence aspects of aging, such as the density and strength of our bones and their resistance to fractures. (Women can enter menopause with stronger bones if they build them well early in life by eating a healthy diet and maintaining normal body weight; by not smoking and not consuming alcohol excessively; by getting adequate vitamin D from sun exposure and supplements; and by doing the right kind and amount of exercise.)

These lifestyle measures may sound simple, but they are profoundly effective. Here are just a handful of the many, many examples. I present them merely as an introduction to the power of prevention.

Preventive Benefits of
Dietary Modification

- Risks of cancer, heart disease, stroke, diabetes, and many other chronic diseases can be reduced with an adequate intake of fruits and vegetables, but only 11 percent of Americans meet the United States Department of Agriculture (USDA) guidelines for these foods. In one study, people who consumed vegetables six to seven days per week had a 54 percent lower risk of stroke (the third highest cause of death) than those who ate vegetables zero to two days per week.

- Studies indicate that a diet high in fruits and vegetables and low in salt and saturated fat helps prevent cardiovascular disease by normalizing blood pressure.

- Many fruits and vegetables contain phytonutrients that help prevent cancers of the lung, breast, colon, and prostate.

- A diet rich in the flavonoids found in tea, chocolate, onions, and other foods lowers the risk of heart disease by up to 20 percent.

- Cruciferous vegetables such as broccoli, cabbage, and kale lower the risk of breast and other forms of cancer and help counter the damage done by smoking, resulting in fewer cancers of the head and neck.

- Compounds in onions and garlic inhibit the growth of breast cancer cells and can cut the risk of stomach cancer by half and colorectal cancer by two-thirds.

- The phytoestrogens in soy appear to lower the incidence of reproductive and breast cancers in females who eat soy foods regularly before puberty.

- Most cases of type-2 diabetes can be successfully controlled with proper diet and adequate physical activity. In genetically susceptible individuals, type-2 diabetes can be prevented by maintaining normal weight and sensitivity to insulin through attention to diet and physical activity.

Preventive Benefits of Dietary Supplementation

- The nutrient lutein (a carotenoid pigment found in orange and yellow fruits and vegetables) has significant preventive effects on macular degeneration, the leading cause of blindness in adults.

- The B complex of vitamins has a number of preventive properties. Ingestion of B12 and B6 has been shown to reduce failure rates after heart surgery. One study indicated that lowering levels of the amino acid homocysteine by taking B12 and folic acid reduced the risk of heart disease by 16 percent and stroke by 24 percent. Niacin (B3) is a proven therapy to lower serum lipid levels.
- Selenium may significantly reduce the risk of prostate cancer, particularly when used in conjunction with other prostate-protective nutrients, including vitamin D and fish oil.
- Vitamin C has a wide range of preventive actions. It helps prevent cancer by blocking effects of carcinogens. It inhibits the oxidation of LDL cholesterol by about 75 percent and so helps prevent heart disease. It helps prevent sun damage to the skin by destroying free radicals. It aids in the control of *Helicobacter pylori* (*H. pylori*), the bacterium associated with peptic ulcers and stomach cancer. In a twenty-year study, vitamin C was shown to significantly decrease the risk of gout.
- Vitamin D is vital to proper immune

function, which is pivotally important in disease prevention, but many people are deficient in it. Vitamin D not only strengthens our defenses but also prevents some autoimmune disorders, particularly multiple sclerosis (which is much more common in America's northern states) and type-1 diabetes. Recently, it has been shown to offer strong protection against some of the most common and dangerous types of cancers, including those of the breast, prostate, pancreas, and colon. Some research indicates that it may reduce risk of these cancers by 50 percent or more. We have long known that vitamin D builds bone strength, reducing the risk of osteoporosis and hip fractures in the elderly.

Preventive Benefits of Exercise

- Lack of exercise and poor diet are the two most significant contributors to obesity, the greatest single cause of illness in our society.
- Compared to those who are sedentary, females who exercise regularly between the ages of twelve and thirty-five have an estimated 23 percent lower risk of pre-menopausal breast cancer, which

accounts for one-fourth of all breast cancer cases.

- Exercise decreases arthritic pain and dysfunction by strengthening muscles around joints, reducing stress on the joints, and reducing stiffness.
- Regular exercise appears to significantly improve survival rates among people with cancer.
- Exercise both prevents and alleviates depression, often as significantly as treatment with drugs. It can also help relieve anxiety.
- Aerobic exercise improves the function of the lungs and heart, resulting in increased resistance to heart disease and chronic obstructive pulmonary disease.
- Exercise is pivotally important in the prevention and treatment of diabetes, due to its effects on body fat and metabolism.

Preventive Benefits of Stress Management
- Engaging in relaxation techniques, including meditation, has been clearly shown to lower blood pressure, improve heart function, enhance digestion, produce calming brain waves, reduce the symptoms of premenstrual

syndrome, boost immune function, and improve milk flow in lactating women.

- In a study of people with a variety of chronic conditions and diseases, patients who practiced meditation experienced less pain, anxiety, and depression than those who did not.
- Stress reduction is closely associated with a lower risk of heart disease.
- Short-term psychotherapy focused on stress management has been shown to reduce health-care costs by up to 20 percent over a period of several years.
- Stress has a significant impact on the incidence and severity of headaches, asthma, chronic pain, arthritis, heart disease, fibromyalgia, and chronic fatigue syndrome.
- Getting enough sleep of good quality promotes health. Sleeping fewer than seven hours per night has been shown to increase the risk of high blood pressure, diabetes, weight gain, and hardening of the arteries. People who sleep restlessly for more than one-half hour per night are estimated to have five times the risk of minor illnesses, such as colds, compared to those who sleep soundly.

These are but a few of the preventive measures that can exert extraordinary influence over our susceptibility to disease and the way we age. But the most important steps we can take are to avoid smoking and obesity. These two risk factors alone account for almost 1 million American deaths every year out of the 2.5 million who die of all causes combined.

THE HIGH RISK OF SMOKING

Tobacco in the form of cigarettes is as addictive as crack cocaine. Tobacco smoking is the most common preventable cause of cancer in our society; it is also a major risk factor for cardiovascular and respiratory disease. Our attempts to contain its potential for harm have been hailed as a public health triumph, but I consider them only partially successful. In the 1960s, 42 percent of American adults smoked, compared to 20 percent in 2005. That's the good news. The bad news is that the decrease has slowed. Smoking is increasingly concentrated in lower socioeconomic groups, and it still accounts for 430,000 premature deaths per year. In some groups (Native Americans and African-American men) the rates of smoking are going up. We have used laws, taxes, litigation, and education to try to dissuade Americans from smoking, but without the social consensus needed to effect a cultural change, none of these mechanisms can be as effective as we'd like them to be.

The modern cigarette is an American invention that dates back only to the 1860s. Before then, tobacco was too harsh to allow smokers to inhale nicotine deeply or often enough to make their brains dependent on it. Two developments changed that: the introduction of a milder tobacco variety and a new method of processing its leaves that made the smoke less irritating. Most people who tried the new cigarettes became addicted smokers, and the tobacco companies had an ideal product — one that sold without effort, created customers for life, and made them fortunes.

The importance of tobacco in our country's economy has skewed American attitudes toward it, including our assessment of its effect on health. Soon after Columbus brought the plant back from the New World, the use of tobacco spread throughout the Old World, and governments realized that it could be a valuable resource. They taxed it and took control of its distribution. By the 1800s, tobacco was a major source of revenue in the United States. When the tobacco industry began selling highly addictive cigarettes, its growth exploded. It was this success that was chiefly responsible for the South's economic recovery after the Civil War.

Earlier in American history, alcoholism was far more common than it is today. Men, women, and even children would start drinking whiskey in the morning and be drunk on the sidewalks at night. This epidemic gradually declined, however, as the culture surrounding strong forms of alcohol changed. A process of social learning about acceptable ways to drink curbed epidemic drunkenness. A similar process could help us reduce the number of Americans addicted to tobacco.

Tobacco, though, is even more economically and politically ingrained into our society than alcohol. Tobacco leaves decorate the columns on the Senate side of the U.S. Capitol in recognition of their contribution to the national economy. For much of our history no one could become president of our country without the support of the tobacco industry. Powerful economic forces still impede the public health effort to reduce smoking.

The Toll of Smoking

- Smoking is responsible for approximately one in every five deaths in America.
- Smokers die an average of thirteen to fourteen years younger than nonsmokers.
- Smokers develop coronary heart disease two to four times more frequently than nonsmokers.
- Lung cancer — much of it smoking related — is the most common fatal cancer among American men and women combined and is the most common cause of cancer death in the world.
- Smoking is even worse for women than men. Female smokers are three times more likely than male smokers to have lung cancer or heart disease. Lung cancer has increased among women by five times in the past twenty years and now kills more women than breast cancer. Women who smoke are six times more likely to have a heart attack than nonsmoking women, and women who smoke and use birth control pills are twenty times more likely than nonsmokers to have heart disease. Women who smoke have higher rates

of depression than nonsmokers and more facial wrinkles at a younger age.

- Children who smoke before age seventeen are 2.7 times more likely to develop multiple sclerosis than nonsmoking young people. A study of MS patients revealed that 32 percent were early smokers. (The great majority of tobacco addicts began smoking as teens.)
- Smoking accounts for up to half of all cases of bladder cancer, but three-fourths of all people with bladder cancer did not know it was a risk factor.
- Chronic Obstructive Pulmonary Disease (COPD), including emphysema, is America's fourth leading cause of death, accounting for more deaths than diabetes and twice as many as Alzheimer's. It kills more people than all accidents combined. Smoking is the major risk factor.
- Smoking also causes cancers of the larynx, mouth and throat, esophagus, kidney, pancreas, colon, cervix, and stomach, as well as acute myeloid leukemia.

Until fairly recently Americans regarded

tobacco as a good thing, and our government saw no reason to discourage its use. (It included cigarettes in the emergency rations of soldiers right up to the 1970s.) Smoking may have annoyed nonusers, but few thought it was harmful. Many people believed that it improved concentration and the productivity of workers. Once the social taboo against women smoking dissolved in the early 1900s, women took up the habit enthusiastically; it helped many of them curb eating and weight gain. In fact, smoking was in high fashion in our country for much of the twentieth century. Smokers appeared glamorous, sexy, and a tad rebellious, characteristics that enticed many young Americans to join their ranks. Movie stars and other celebrities smoked. Successful people smoked. Athletes smoked. Intellectuals smoked. Cigarette makers played up these themes in ads that targeted young people, their future customers. They knew that most young people who tried cigarettes would not stop using them and that if people didn't smoke before age twenty, there was a 90 percent chance they never would.

Even doctors smoked. As late as the 1950s, doctors appeared in ads for cigarettes, giving assurances that certain brands were less irritating or even good for the throat. Not until the mid-1980s did the American Medical Association, under pressure from members, divest itself of its large holdings of tobacco stock.

Once a more accurate understanding of the nature and risks of tobacco addiction grew in the medical community, concerned experts started campaigns to fight it in order to prevent the diseases it caused. The antismoking movement has relied on a variety of strategies, such as banning smoking in public places and restricting tobacco sales to minors, taxing tobacco to make it less affordable (especially for young people), pressuring the tobacco industry to put health warnings on products and drop some kinds of advertising, launching massive educational efforts to make people aware of the dangers of smoking, and supporting much-publicized class-action and individual lawsuits on behalf of people harmed or killed by tobacco-related diseases. We have seen the demographics of smoking change as a result — down in some groups and up in others. But too many Americans still smoke, and our health-care system is left to deal with the consequences.

Analysts have tried to evaluate the effect that each of these antismoking strategies has had in reducing the incidence of smoking and changing its demographics. They discount the influence of lawsuits against tobacco companies, which have had mixed success, and of restrictions on advertising, which have inspired companies to find ways of getting around them (such as using more print ads and billboards instead of television and radio commercials). Most effective, they think, have been informational initiatives that warn about health risks and the added taxes on cigarettes, which tend to deter young people from buying them.

Reducing smoking in our population to a level we can live with will require a comprehensive society-wide effort. Our success so far has been limited for the following reasons.

- Although smoking has gone out of fashion in some subgroups, it has not in others. Too many Americans still think smoking makes you look more adventurous, sexy, or interesting. In particular, too many youngsters see it as a sign of maturity or a convenient way to express rebellion. And too many women rely on it to control their weight.
- Advertising and the media still portray

smokers in ways that lead young people to try cigarettes. I see more smoking on movie screens today than I did ten years ago. The images are powerfully seductive.

- Warnings on cigarette labels about long-term health risks of lung cancer and emphysema mean little to teenagers. A more effective warning might be: "Most people who try cigarettes become addicted users. Nicotine in this form is more addictive than heroin."
- Despite all the pressure on them, the tobacco companies still have undue influence on government and policy. They have bought and controlled some of our most senior senators and representatives, and have relentlessly fought the antismoking movement. When bans on smoking in public places were first proposed, tobacco companies tried to convince smokers that a constitutionally guaranteed right to free expression was at stake.
- Although we have made tobacco products more expensive, they remain widely available — in all convenience stores, pharmacies, and supermarkets.

These are big obstacles, but, unquestionably, they can be overcome. Of paramount importance is education to raise awareness of the nature and consequences of tobacco addiction. *There would be no antismoking movement if people had not become aware of the health hazards of that addiction.* Until people were informed about the dangers of breathing secondhand smoke, for example, few of them cared enough to do anything about smoking in public. Many people underestimated the harm of secondhand smoke, which is now clearly documented. (In Pueblo, Colorado, for example, a ban on public smoking resulted within three years in a 41 percent decrease in hospitalizations for heart attacks.) In this and other battles against smoking, the political will that was necessary to overcome corporate power and its influence on government was totally a product of raised awareness.

And how was awareness raised? I would say entirely as the result of medical research and the informational initiatives of health professionals, including public health workers. Further progress in preventing our people from becoming tobacco addicts and minimizing the harm that tobacco causes us individually and as a nation will be totally dependent on *continued* and *better* efforts of health professionals and public health workers. Here is what I would like to see.

Strategies for Reducing Smoking in America

- A total ban on advertising of *any* kind of tobacco product.
- A ban on glamorous depictions of smoking in movies and other media.
- Media campaigns to encourage more people to view smoking negatively, such as realistically portraying it as a habit of less attractive, less successful people. This will help speed its going out of fashion. These portrayals should focus on the extreme addictive potential of cigarettes. We have played up the future risks of chronic disease but have largely ignored the immediate danger of addiction.
- Elimination of smoking from all public places. This has already been achieved on a national level in the tiny country of Bhutan, which has also banned sales of tobacco, requiring addicts to import it and pay a stiff tax. Norway recently imposed a national ban on smoking in public, and other countries will probably follow.
- Increased restrictions on sales of to-

bacco, resulting in its eventual removal from convenience stores, pharmacies, and supermarkets. San Francisco has already passed an order banning the sale of tobacco products at pharmacies, although the Walgreen Company, with fifty-two outlets in the city, has asked a California state court to overturn the law as "anticompetitive and unconstitutional."
- Subsidies to tobacco farmers, to help them switch to other crops.

The collective will to achieve these goals will require a consensus in our diverse society that tobacco is an addictive and dangerous drug, that we would all be better off if our country were free of it, that smoking in public is intolerable, and that tobacco use is inconsistent with healthy living. Our institutions of public health must take responsibility for creating that consensus by vigorously gathering and disseminating accurate information about the impact of tobacco use on health. I have strong faith in the ability of people to change their ways of living if they have access to truthful information that makes sense to them. We should proceed in the movement against tobacco addiction in much the same way that we steer the entire movement against all bad health habits — with education instead of coercion — as we create a new culture of health.

Cultural change is hard, but it happens. For example, I remember clearly how my own resistance to wearing seat belts disappeared. Early on, like many people, I regarded them as a silly inconvenience. "Buckle up" was the sort of message I got from parents and teachers and that I ignored. But one day I was driving a rough road with a close friend, someone I did not in any way regard as "parental." He got me to stop and put my seat belt on. Then he said, "Now you look as if you're ready to *really* drive a car." Shortly afterward I learned that most deaths and severe injuries in auto accidents resulted from people being thrown from their cars. I hadn't known that, and it made sense. Together with my friend's advice, it got me to buckle up whenever I got in a car — a good habit instead of a bad one.

Car wrecks kill about 42,000 people each year and injure 4 million, so it would be foolish to argue that wearing seat belts is not relevant to lifestyle medicine and prevention.

The saga of improving American lives by

getting people to use seat belts has a number of familiar themes. When safety experts first called for their use, car manufacturers refused to install them as standard equipment, because they didn't want to bear the expense and thought the discussion of safety would lessen our love for cars. (Later, they also resisted air bags, despite overwhelming evidence that they saved lives.) Acceptance of seat belts was the result of informational campaigns, laws, and incentives from insurance companies, resulting in an increase of use from 11 percent in 1981 to 68 percent in 1997 (and 91 percent in California).

What makes me most optimistic is not the effect of legal sanctions but, once again, the power of education and social learning: a change in our culture. Many times I have heard children tell grown-ups to put on seat belts. These kids are part of a new culture in which not wearing seat belts is unthinkable. I became part of that culture through the influence of a friend and an exposure to factual information. The emerging new system of American health care must *create a culture* in which our other most destructive health choices become unthinkable: smoking, being sedentary, and eating low-quality foods. If this does not happen, we will waste even more money and effort on drastic interventions while American health outcomes continue to deteriorate and our country sinks under debt.

OBESITY:
OUR GREATEST OBSTACLE
TO DISEASE PREVENTION

Rampant obesity has now emerged as the gravest threat to American public health, although we have barely begun to experience its full medical consequences and fiscal burdens. If you have any doubt about how much heavier Americans are now than they used to be, I urge you to look at images from the 1930s or 1940s. I just finished watching the excellent PBS documentary series *The War,* the story of World War II, which includes many crowd scenes of our civilian workers and armed forces. There are virtually *no* fat people in those crowds. Americans then didn't know as much about nutrition as we do, didn't buy "health foods," and ate a lot of things that health-conscious people today avoid. What happened?

Most of us are less active than our parents and grandparents. We walk less and spend more time sitting in front of televisions and computers. Physical education has been dropped from many public schools, a casualty of funding cuts. Maybe more of us overeat to satisfy emotional needs. But I think the main driver of the obesity epidemic, even more than how *much* we eat, is *what* we now eat, because food has changed greatly in the past fifty years. Our grandparents would not recognize much of the food that Americans eat today.

Most of the obesity we see around us, including the childhood obesity that is so alarming, is the result of a disorder rooted in a disturbed function of insulin, the master hormone that regulates the body's distribution, use, and storage of caloric energy. The disorder is called *metabolic syndrome.* Predisposition to it is inherited, and the multiple genes responsible for it are very frequent in our population. Their frequency is a legacy of evolution that probably helped our distant ancestors survive famine. But those genes were just as widespread in our population in the 1940s. Since then, unfortunately, interactions between genes and changed eating patterns have made our cells resistant to insulin. Insulin resistance is the root imbalance in metabolic syndrome.

The most significant change in American eating patterns since World War II is our greatly increased consumption of the processed, refined, and manufactured food that has displaced whole, natural food in our diet. Few families today cook meals from scratch (or even sit down to meals together). Instead, they mostly buy and consume manufactured food, much of it made with ingredients that are new to human diets, such as highly refined vegetable oils and starches, high-fructose corn syrup, and innumerable additives. Modern food technology has drastically altered the foods that nature provides, all too often reducing their nutritive qualities and increasing their potential for harm. The net result has been horrific. Here is just a sample of the innumerable ways that obesity is undermining American health and hobbling attempts at disease prevention.

The Toll of Obesity

- Obesity is linked to more than thirty medical conditions, including all of the most destructive chronic degenerative diseases: heart disease, stroke, cancer, diabetes, age-related dementia, and osteoarthritis.
- Cancer is closely linked to obesity. Obesity is the greatest risk factor for colorectal cancer among women, as well as a major one for endometrial (uterine) cancer. Women who gain

more than 45 pounds after age eighteen are twice as likely to develop breast cancer. Obesity is strongly associated with cancer of the esophagus — risk increases as weight increases — and it accounts for an estimated 21 percent of renal cell (kidney) cancer. It is also one of the primary risk factors for prostate cancer.

- Obesity is very closely associated with heart disease and stroke. An estimated 46 percent of all obese adults have high blood pressure, one of the major risk factors for cardiovascular disease. Over 75 percent of deaths related to high blood pressure occur in people who are obese. Obesity is intimately associated with diabetes. Up to 90 percent of all people with type-2 diabetes are overweight or obese. Obesity increases insulin resistance and worsens metabolic syndrome, which are the predecessors of type-2 diabetes. Obesity also decreases the effectiveness of medications used to treat diabetes.
- Obesity is a predictor of osteoarthritis, particularly of the knees, and contributes to degeneration of the joints in the hips, knees, and lower back. It severely aggravates joint pain, as well

as pain from other chronic medical conditions.

- Obesity is now believed to contribute to asthma; 75 percent of patients who visit the emergency room for asthma are obese.
- Obesity increases the risk of end-stage renal (kidney) disease by seven times and is an independent risk factor for the development of progressive liver disease, including cirrhosis and chronic hepatitis.
- Obesity contributes to a wide range of other disorders and conditions, including sleep apnea, postpartum depression and clinical depression, cervical pain, back pain, hiatal hernia, pancreatitis, urinary stress incontinence, gastroesophageal reflux, endocrine abnormalities, skin problems, heel spurs, and immune dysfunction.

How We Are Trapped

When I go into convenience stores in this country, I have a hard time finding real food or food with no questionable ingredients. If I'm lucky, I can get a jar of dry-roasted peanuts without monosodium glutamate (MSG). Otherwise, it's frozen bright blue slush swirling in a dispenser, shelves of soft drinks, and arrays of snack foods with multitudes of ingredients in fine print. Many of these foods — chips, pretzels, breads, cookies, pastries — are high in quick-digesting carbohydrates that are potent triggers of insulin resistance and metabolic syndrome. I don't have much more success in supermarkets unless I stick to the periphery, mostly the produce counters. As soon as I venture into the interior aisles, I see only the same processed stuff.

The products that dominate American convenience stores, supermarkets, fast-food restaurants, and kitchen tables are low-quality foods, less nutritious and less health-ful than the whole foods people ate when I was growing up, which were much closer to their natural state. They are also ultimately less satisfying even if they offer immediate gratification. I see Americans eating more and more and enjoying it less and less. That is why so much mindless eating goes on all day long in our society (while driving and watching television and movies) and why portions have grown so large — Big Gulps of soft drinks and buckets of popcorn, for example. Food in France and Italy, by contrast, is of much higher quality; people take time to enjoy it and get much more pleasure from it. As a result, they are satisfied with smaller portions, eat less frequently than we do, and have much less obesity even though they love such foods as cheese, bread, and pasta that we consider fattening. Unfortunately, wherever in the world people develop preferences for American-type fast food and processed food, rates of obesity go up. Predictable health consequences soon follow.

If American food is responsible for American obesity, what can we do about it? Serious proposals have been made for a "sin tax" on junk food and fast food, for an "overweight" surcharge on airline fares, and for a health-care tax on the obese. Would any of these work? How can we formulate effective policy to improve American eating habits?

This is a harder problem than curbing smoking or alcohol abuse or getting people to wear seat belts. But we must tackle it. Here are my thoughts on strategies for change:

Ending the Obesity Epidemic
- Most Americans have never heard of metabolic syndrome; relatively few understand its prevalence and relationship to food choices. We have to change

this. Education is our best hope for prevention and treatment of obesity.

- Relatively few of our health professionals have any working knowledge of obesity. Most physicians are poorly educated in nutrition. Many doctors, registered dieticians, and other experts continue to recommend low-fat diets for weight loss or tell patients to cut calories and exercise more, ignoring the critical importance of the kinds of foods they eat. Correcting the professional knowledge gap is as important as informing the public.

- Most of our hospitals and medical centers serve the worst kinds of modern American food, so that after a consultation about weight loss, a family can go right to the in-house fast-food restaurant for a meal guaranteed to accelerate the development of insulin resistance. Fast food has no place in these settings. The food in health-care facilities should taste good as well as exemplify good nutritional principles. It should inspire patients, families, visitors, and staff to make better food choices.

- People eat what is available and what is affordable, and the most available and affordable food in our country makes many people fat and increases their long-term health risks. We have to make unhealthy food expensive and healthy food much cheaper.

- Any discussion of restricting the production and marketing of harmful foods gets shouted down as unacceptable interference with American business. Sorry, but this discussion is all-important. When it comes to food, the free market is doing us in. Big food companies say they are just giving people what they want, but we have to persuade or force them to take responsibility for making better products and changing people's tastes. Accomplishing this may depend on grass-roots movements (such as the ones that got soft drink vending machines out of many schools), legislation (such as the bans on trans fats), boycotts, and other forms of public and political pressure.
- Government inertia in this area is due to ignorance and, I'm afraid, to the all-too-common tendency to protect private gain rather than public good. The tobacco lobby slowed government support for the antismoking movement for years, and auto makers delayed legisla-

tion requiring cars to have air bags. Today, it's the giant food corporations that are calling the shots on food policy. We must neutralize corporate influence on government and exert rightful direction of policy.

- The health-care community has been of little help in redirecting policy because it is uninformed, asleep, and politically inept. The Farm Bill (which should be called the Food and Farm Bill so that more of us would pay attention to it) is a massive package of legislation that is redrafted every five years. It affects our food choices, our agricultural practices, and the health of our environment. As I wrote previously, the crop subsidies provided by this bill make unhealthy foods cheaper than healthy ones and play a large part in the obesity of our population. Big corporations shape Farm Bill subsidies through their powerful lobbies. The health-care consequences of those subsidies cost us vastly more than the corporations gain, but this fact is never mentioned in congressional Farm Bill debates. The health-care community has made almost no effort to oppose the agribusiness lobby. It must do so.

- Because children are at greatest risk, we must concentrate our obesity prevention efforts on them. Again, I believe that education is our best resource. I have seen good messages on public television about food that educate kids to see garishly colored breakfast cereals and snacks as unnatural and scary rather than attractive and help them perceive fresh vegetables as powerhouses of energy. We have made minimal use of innovative forms of education to counteract the influence of harmful advertising on kids. Let's change that today.
- We must protect the poor, who are at higher risk. The density of fast-food restaurants is greater in poor neighborhoods, and the quality of foods available in stores is lower. If you have ever gone into a grocery store on an Indian reservation, you know why metabolic syndrome is so prevalent and so devastating among Native Americans. Yes, they may be more genetically prone to it, but changed dietary preferences are mainly to blame, and those are a function of what foods are available. In July 2008 the Los Angeles City Council voted unanimously to place a morato-

rium on new fast-food restaurants in an impoverished area of the city where fast-food chains have proliferated, along with obesity. The vote stirred intense controversy, and the California Restaurant Association announced plans to fight the move. No surprise there. I welcome this kind of legislation if only as a sign that officials are thinking about the causes of epidemic obesity in new ways.

- We must also do everything we can, of course, to promote physical activity in our population. I applaud former CDC director Dr. Julie Gerberding for calling for more bike paths and pedestrian walkways in cities. We must pressure governments to restore funding to schools for physical education. We must also work for greater funding of public education in general so that school districts can refuse offers of money from fast-food chains and soft drink makers in exchange for marketing access to schoolchildren.

These are the kinds of challenges we face, and these are the actions I endorse, along with asking that Americans take greater personal responsibility for their own health.

Out with the Old Preventive Medicine and in with the New

What goes on in our country under the banner of "preventive medicine" causes me profound dismay. There is currently a specialty with that name recognized by the AMA. To qualify for it, a physician must complete a one-year internship and a residency of at least two years (including completion of a master's degree in public health), do a year of practice, and pass board exams. Preventive medicine became a designated specialty in 1948, and today some two thousand men and women are members of the American College of Preventive Medicine. This is not sufficient. There are twenty-three times more psychiatrists and sixty-five times more internists, in part because prevention specialists make less money and have less status.

The stated goals of the American College of Preventive Medicine are laudable — education about causation of illness, research on lifestyle factors that influence disease risks, and lobbying for a healthier environment, for example — but in practice the influence of these efforts on American health care has been minimal. We must transform preventive medicine into a vigorous, influential field with a strong clinical arm. We could start by attracting more practitioners, using subsidized training and other financial incentives, and giving the whole field a new image, perhaps with the help of marketing and public relations experts. The money this would cost would be a pittance compared to what it would save.

But I'm afraid there is a more fundamental concern here: Preventive medicine as it exists today has not been terribly successful, and that fact, more than its lack of glamour and low wages, seems to me the main reason for the field's weakness. We have thrown a great deal of money and effort at preventing cancer, sexually transmitted diseases, drug abuse, and many other terrible health problems without much to show for it. I see no quick and easy fix for this record of failure, because it is our fundamental ways of thinking about the causation and prevention of disease that are holding us back and that need to change. Just as we must transform interventional medicine, breaking its dependence on costly high-tech methods of managing disease, we must also devise a new paradigm of preventive medicine.

I have argued that interventional medicine must recognize complexity; so, too, must

243

preventive medicine. For example, because it is well known that sun exposure causes skin cancer, the conventional approach is to get people to avoid the sun or use sunscreen. But being out in the sun is also very good for us, physically and mentally. It is the best way to get the "sunshine vitamin," vitamin D, which is actually a hormone produced in the skin by the action of ultraviolet (UV) light. We have vitamin D receptors in all our tissues; it is a basic regulator of cell growth and development and one of our most important defenses against cancer and other chronic diseases. It is almost impossible to get enough of it from food sources, and if you live anywhere north of 34 degrees latitude — about that of Atlanta, Georgia — the sun is too low in the sky from October through March to give you enough UV rays to make what you need. If you regularly apply sunscreen, you won't make enough vitamin D even during the summer months, no matter where you live.

As new information about the vital importance of adequate vitamin D for optimum health has emerged, more doctors have begun to measure blood levels in patients. They are finding that many Americans are severely deficient, and we have good evidence that vitamin D deficiency is associated with increased risks of many forms of cancer and autoimmune diseases. You can remedy and prevent vitamin D deficiency by taking it as a dietary supplement. (I take 2,000 IU a day with a fat-containing meal to ensure absorption and recommend that to everyone.) But the best way to get it is to go out in the sun. There is no danger of getting too much vitamin D that way, and sunlight also increases the number of vitamin D receptors in the skin. We lose those receptors as we age, and taking supplements does not restore them.

Daily exposure to bright sunlight also optimizes cyclic secretion of melatonin, the neurotransmitter that controls biorhythms and influences immunity and hormonal function. Time in the sun boosts mood and helps prevent depression.

But by relying on linear thinking, dermatologists and other medical experts have come to the conclusion that the sun is a threat to health, plain and simple, and have persuaded many of us to regard it as an enemy. By telling women that the sun will make them look old and wrinkled before their time, beauty experts reinforce that view. The sunscreen industry is booming. (It is also a major funder of the American Academy of Dermatology.)

If the main concern is skin cancer, we should keep in mind that the common forms of it are easily detected and cured. Only melanoma, a relatively rare malignancy, is as serious a threat to general health and life as the much more frequent cancers linked to vitamin D deficiency. A more useful view is that solar radiation can both increase and decrease cancer risks through a complex environmental interaction involving many variables, including differences in genes, biochemistry, and lifestyle. Estimating how many cases of potentially deadly cancers would be prevented if more people received the right amount, intensity, and regularity of sunlight — versus how many more cases of potentially deadly melanoma might occur — would be a useful first step toward formulating sounder recommendations.

And even that estimation would only scratch the surface of the matter, because it ignores the other positive effects of sunlight and because we know so little about *all* the ways that the sun affects us. The challenge is to achieve balance with an environmental influence that can both harm us and help us.

The Old Way: Prevention with Pharmaceuticals

I have heard more than one cardiologist state that statins are so effective, they should be added to the water supply. Forget it. I agree that, to date, statins are the most effective cholesterol-lowering medications developed, and I fully support their use in selected patients. But I regard unbridled enthusiasm for them as preventive agents to be unfounded, another product of the obsolete model of preventive medicine still in vogue and a stunning example of disregard for the complexity of disease causation.

What we want to prevent are heart attacks, because they are common killers in our population and are associated with other cardiovascular diseases whose management costs us lots of money. We know that heart attack risk is increased in those who smoke, have high blood pressure, eat typical Western diets, are inactive, and tend to rage when frustrated — habits and traits that can be modified. Genetic influences are also significant — and complex.

Elevated serum cholesterol is but one element in this mix of risk factors. Half of those who suffer first heart attacks have normal levels of serum cholesterol. That fact alone should give pause to the statins-in-the-water-supply folks. Moreover, the effectiveness of statins is very focused: They lower one type of cholesterol: low-density lipoprotein (LD), the "bad cholesterol" that can adhere to the lining of arteries, build up, and eventually restrict blood flow. They do not raise levels of high-density lipoprotein (HDL), the good fraction that protects arteries from this kind of damage. They also fail to lower levels of fats (triglycerides) circulating in the blood. These are changes we would like to see in those at risk. The more we study the relationship between serum lipids (fats) and cardiovascular disease, the more complexity we find. There are types and subtypes of LDL and HDL and variations in the size and density of their particles. Some serum lipid profiles indicate more risk than others. We would like to be able to modify them — for example, reduce the number of small, dense LDL particles and increase the number of larger, fluffier ones. Statins do not enable us to do this. They are a crude intervention, just as measurements of total serum cholesterol or LDL are crude indicators of cardiovascular health.

And remember that even lipid abnormalities are but one of many factors contributing to heart attack risk. Enthusiasm for and widespread use of statins have diverted attention from addressing modifiable risk factors such as diet, lack of physical activity, stress, and uncontrolled anger. Many doctors who put patients on these drugs to reduce risk of heart attack feel they have fulfilled their preventive responsibilities. It doesn't matter what patients eat or how they handle stress; it has all been taken care of with the prescription.

In our drug-happy society, prescribing medications is increasingly the mainstay of preventive medicine. We identify ever more "preconditions," such as prehypertension, prediabetes, and osteopenia (bone weakness), and then put patients on long-term drug therapy to block progression to full-blown conditions and their damaging effects. Is this a cost-effective and efficient strategy? The pharmaceutical companies produce evidence that it is, but much of that evidence is questionable.

Drugs are compared to placebos in randomized controlled trials in order to determine their efficacy at reducing risk of bad outcomes. The "relative risk reduction" as reported in medical journals often looks impressive: Statin therapy, for example, reduces risk of heart attack by 36 percent.

But statistics can be misleading.

In evaluating whether an intervention is worth it, we should not pay much attention to the relative risk reduction measured by comparing the incidence of bad outcomes (heart attacks) in a group of patients taking a statin to the incidence of bad outcomes in a control group. Much more relevant is the number needed to treat (NNT), a fairly recent innovation in medical thinking. The NNT tells us how many patients we would need to put on statin therapy in order to prevent one heart attack in a certain time interval.

Here is an actual example of how it is calculated: A manufacturer-sponsored study addressed the benefit of 10 milligrams daily of Lipitor (atorvastatin) in patients with high blood pressure but no previous cardiovascular disease. The benefit the investigators had in mind was prevention of heart attacks. The trial ran for 3 1/4 years, and during this period the relative risk of heart attack was reduced by 36 percent. That is, there were 36 percent fewer heart attacks in those on Lipitor than those on the placebo. Sounds great, doesn't it? But because the total number of heart attacks in the study group was small, the absolute risk reduction (the rate in the control subgroup [2.67

percent] minus the rate in the treated subgroup [1.65 percent]) was much smaller, only 1.02 percent. The number needed to treat is the inverse of this last figure: 1 divided by 1.02 percent, or 99.7. This means that based on the results of this study, you would have to give Lipitor to one hundred people for 3 1/4 years in order to prevent one heart attack.

Lipitor, like other statins, is expensive — about $900 a year for the lowest daily dose of 10 milligrams. (Many patients take much more.) It is one of the best-selling pharmaceutical products, generating up to $10 billion a year for Pfizer, its manufacturer. Also, like other statins, it can cause adverse effects, some serious. Prescribing it to one hundred patients to prevent one heart attack certainly benefits Pfizer and certainly adds to the cost of American health care, but I don't think it does a lot for American health, which is why I'll never join the chorus of physicians who advocate putting statins in our water supply in the name of preventive medicine.

The same kind of analysis leaves me unconvinced of the wisdom of other popular uses of drugs for disease prevention. Let me take you through one more case: the vogue for starting women on bone-building drugs to prevent osteoporosis, a common and serious disease. We lose bone mass and strength as we age, women sooner than men, because menopause in midlife removes the protective effect of estrogen. (Levels of sex hormones in men remain high until old age.) In osteoporosis, bones lose calcium, becoming less dense and less strong. This is serious because it greatly increases the risk of hip fractures, a major cause of disability and death in older people. (When people become immobile after a fracture, their breathing is impaired, and they are at high risk for pneumonia.) It is medically fashionable today to diagnose "osteopenia" in young and middle-aged women by bone scans. Osteopenia means diminished calcification of bones, and women are told it is the precondition leading to osteoporosis, making them anxious and willing to go along with the preventive measure of taking — long-term — drugs such as Fosamax and Actonel, which are heavily promoted as bone-building agents.

These drugs, in a class called bisphosphonates, are not benign. They can harm the esophagus and stomach, and occasionally cause death of the jawbone (a reaction noted first not by prescribing physicians but by oral surgeons who saw it in their patients on the drugs). Bisphosphonates are also expensive (up to several hundred dollars a month), and while they improve the appearance of bone on scans, the bone they build may not be normal bone. I do not think we know enough about their long-term effects to be using them as casually as we are.

But putting aside the possibility of harm, the main question here is whether this measure is worth it. What we want to prevent are hip fractures in older women. Should we even be screening so many younger women for early changes in bone density? Is osteopenia a legitimate medical concern? And this is the big question: How many hip fractures do we, in fact, prevent by putting younger women on these costly drugs? Their manufacturers would have us believe they are smashingly effective. Here's an excerpt from information for doctors on Fosamax: "In postmenopausal women, FOSAMAX is proven to prevent hip fractures. As shown in the . . . studies, FOSAMAX reduced the risk of hip fractures by 63 percent . . . in women with and without prior fractures. Consistent results were shown in study after study. There was an overall 52 percent hip fracture risk reduction in a meta-analysis."

But what does this mean? Drug company

reps quote these figures to physicians, who repeat them to patients, never mentioning that this is relative risk reduction in experimental subjects, with percentages that greatly exaggerate efficacy. The more telling number, as I noted earlier, would be the NNT, the number needed to treat. And once again it turns out to be very large, again in the vicinity of one hundred, making the efficacy of bisphosphonate therapy for prevention of hip fractures look quite modest. The cost-effectiveness of drug treatment for osteopenia, an invented precondition, to prevent the serious health consequences of osteoporosis is, in a word, dismal. This approach has outlived its usefulness. It only adds to our health-care costs and woes — just the opposite of what preventive medicine is supposed to do.

FURTHER FLAWS IN OUR CURRENT SYSTEM OF PREVENTION

Troubling questions even arise about some of our most reasonable-seeming preventive methods, such as immunization, fortification of foods with micronutrients, and diagnostic screening for early, curable forms of disease.

Immunization is one of the greatest advances in modern preventive medicine. It is not without risks, but its benefits almost always outweigh those risks. It is responsible for the disappearance of a number of infectious diseases that caused widespread suffering and premature death in the not-so-distant past. Yet more and more people today, many of them well educated, question the value and safety of immunizations and withhold them from their children. Why? Because they have exaggerated fears of adverse reactions to vaccines, believe misinformation about their causing autism, buy into the nonsensical teaching of homeopaths that childhood illnesses such as measles and mumps are necessary for strong immunity and good health in later life, think of vaccines as toxins injected into the body, and reject them along with other "unnatural" methods of conventional medicine. Others argue that we start to vaccinate children too early in life or give too many vaccines at once.

More and more Americans hold these ideas because more and more Americans are discontented with conventional medicine. Some of that discontent is legitimate, but in this case it is misdirected. Maybe we should think about modifying our methods and schedules of immunization to further reduce risk and improve outcomes and compliance. Certainly, we should be constantly trying to improve vaccines to make them safer and more effective. What we really need to understand is how we have failed to educate our citizens about immunization, about its real but limited risks and its very great benefits.

Another example of our flawed system of prevention is the belief that we must fortify foods with vitamins and minerals. Adding micronutrients to foods to prevent disease seems simple — but it isn't. As I mentioned, dietary supplements can be valuable for prevention, but, again, we need to take account of the complexity of their effects before making blanket recommendations in their favor. In early pregnancy a deficiency of folate, a B vitamin, is responsible for neural tube defects (NTD), a class of catastrophic birth defects that include spina bifida. Babies with spina bifida have severe neurological impairment and need costly long-term treatment and management. Folate deficiency is easily prevented by taking folic acid, the synthetic form of the vitamin, as a dietary supplement, but its protective effect occurs so early in embryonic development (in the fourth week) that women may not know they are pregnant. Therefore, any woman who might get pregnant should be on it. How can we ensure that? Many experts called for adding folic acid to common foods, such as flour and other grain products, as a public health measure; others resisted it, arguing that increased folate intake in the general population could have a downside. In particular, it can mask signs of vitamin B12 deficiency, a common problem in the elderly that can also cause serious illness. Proponents of fortification won the day, and in January 1998 the FDA mandated the addition of folic acid to grain products. Since then the incidence of neural tube defects has declined significantly, an apparent public health triumph. New research on folic acid suggests that supplementing the diet with it also reduces risk of colorectal cancer and perhaps other malignancies.

But concerns about what would seem to be a simple preventive measure have not subsided. In fact, they have increased, because even more recent research suggests that consuming more folate might also *stimulate* the development and growth of other types of cancer. Unfortunately, we do not yet know the full story of folate's effects on cell growth and development, we do not know the optimum daily dose, and we do not know how much is too much. The more we look into the matter, the more we are confronted by uncertainty. What if fortification of foods with folic acid turns out to cause more cases of disease than the number of cases of NTD it prevents?

I believe in using dietary supplements, but it is most important to determine the right dosage, because either too little or too much can be ineffective or harmful. I take 400 micrograms of supplemental folic acid as a daily dose and generally recommend that to others, but I don't know whether adding this vitamin to common foods is a good idea.

Another mainstay of conventional prevention is the use of diagnostic screenings to detect early stages of cancer and other diseases, but X-rays and CT scans expose the body to ionizing radiation, which increases cancer risks. We estimate that up to 2 percent of fatal cancers occurring in the next ten to twenty years will directly result from high-tech screenings being done today.

Technology no more represents the future of preventive medicine than it represents the future of interventional medicine. It will have its place. It will save lives. But the only way that we can save a significant number of the approximately 1.7 million people who die each year from preventable illness is with the comprehensive program that I described in this chapter. It won't be easy. But with this approach there is hope. Without it there is only the certainty of more suffering and more expense as American health ebbs and our prosperity declines.

CHAPTER 9
HEALTH PROMOTION:
THE CRITICAL COMPONENT

WHAT IS HEALTH?

According to the World Health Organization, health promotion is the process of enabling people to increase control over and to improve their health. The *American Journal of Health Promotion* defines it as "the science and art of helping people change their lifestyle to move toward a state of optimal health."

All well and good, but I have a big problem with such definitions. A few months ago I spoke to several hundred medical students and residents at a campus of the University of California. My topic was "Integrative Medicine and the Future of Health Care." At the start of my talk I asked the audience a question: What is health? I did not get one satisfactory answer. Mostly I got silence. One person offered, "Well-being," which I dismissed as not saying much. These were physicians and future physicians.

How can we promote health if we do not have a clear sense of what it is? In my experience, many of us think about health only in its absence. When we are sick or injured, we want it restored. One of the most common answers I get when I ask for a definition of it is "absence of disease."

Health is much more interesting and meaningful than the absence of disease. It is no more the absence of disease than wealth is the absence of poverty. Health is a positive state of wholeness and balance in which an organism functions efficiently and interacts smoothly with its environment. Your health depends on innate resilience that allows you to move through life without suffering harm. To illustrate that quality I often suggest the image of a child's knock-down toy with a weighted bottom. Hit the toy however you like, and it comes back to center. Hold it down as long as you like, but as soon as you release it, it comes right back up. The scientific term for the innate resilience of living organisms is *homeostasis* (from Greek roots meaning "standing similar" or "remaining the same"). It denotes the capacity to maintain stability despite changing influences. For example, our internal temperature remains constant over a wide range of environmental temperatures.

Blood flow to vital organs remains constant despite changes in position. Blood sugar is stable even if you don't eat for a time.

If you are healthy, you can interact with germs and not get infections, with allergens and not have allergic reactions, with toxins and not suffer injury. This resilience is not confined to the physical body. If you are in good health, you can also absorb mental and emotional shocks without serious or lasting loss of balance.

"Well-being" does not define health, but it is an attribute of it. In fact, the subjective experience of health is very positive. Healthy people are confident, strong, and aware of their vitality, power, and even their beauty.

My understanding of the relationship between health and beauty grew out of work I did on skin care. A few years ago the CEO of a large cosmetics company asked me to collaborate on the development of innovative skin-care products. She told me that products making antiaging claims were the most successful, but I had just written a book in which I had rejected antiaging as a worthwhile or attainable goal. Instead, I had advised readers to accept the aging process and concentrate on maintaining health at every stage of life. Applying that philosophy to skin care made me focus on ways of supporting the skin's natural defenses. The best way to do that is to give it all the nutrients it needs, particularly essential fatty acids that are deficient in the diets of many. As for topical applications, I came up with the idea of using extracts of mushrooms with anti-inflammatory properties, because low-level, chronic inflammation undermines the health of the skin and other organs.

While working on this project, I came to see that beauty is, in essence, a reflection of health. Animals, for example, advertise their worthiness as potential mates through beauty. Sleek fur and gorgeous plumage are biological signs of good genes and good nourishment. They indicate desirability as a reproductive partner.

People spend a great deal of time, money, and energy on products and services that they think will make them more beautiful and more sexually attractive. It seems to me that a strong selling point for health, one not usually emphasized, is its central contribution to beauty. The health education classes that I sat in from elementary school through high school never mentioned it. Had they done so, they might have been less boring. In the higher grades these classes were taught by gym teachers who presented lackluster material by rote. I would have been eager to learn about optimizing health if I had understood it to be the most powerful way to enhance beauty and sexual attractiveness.

THE NANNY STATE

The medicine of the future must promote health as not just the lack of a negative but as one of the single most positive attributes a person can have. This will not come about by preaching to people. I always felt preached to in my public school health classes. They gave me the same kind of "do this, don't do that" messages I was tired of hearing from parents and other authorities. Telling people to do something or not to do something without helping them understand the reason for it is not simply ineffective but often makes them want to do just the opposite. As I have said, my long resistance to wearing seat belts in cars was in part defiance of authoritarian voices telling me to buckle up. The stated reason was "for safety," which resonated with nothing in my experience and did nothing to change my perception that wearing seat belts was an inconvenience.

Any societal effort that attempts to promote health by telling citizens to make better lifestyle choices confronts a major

264

obstacle. Americans, especially, are not going to put up with a "nanny state" — a government that tells them what to do in the manner of a surrogate parent trying to be excessively protective. This approach is being used in other countries. For example, in Japan health officials measure the waistlines of people over forty and mandate diet counseling for overweight people. If these people fail to lose weight, they can be fined. New Zealand even has a rule that bars obese people from immigrating to the country.

The term "nanny state" is used by both conservatives and liberals to denigrate the political and economic policies of their opponents, and it is frequently used to ridicule efforts to promote health. Witness the title of a book published in 2007: *Nanny State: How Food Fascists, Teetotaling Do-Gooders, Priggish Moralists, and Other Boneheaded Bureaucrats Are Turning America into a Nation of Children.* "Food fascists" is a wonderful epithet for people who tell others what to eat and what not to eat. If some authority figure or government agency were to tell you not to eat products you like because they are bad for you, it would be fair to dismiss that as "food fascism" and continue in your ways.

I recall from long ago an egregious example of nanny state tactics and my own response to them. When I was a college undergraduate, I often drove back and forth between my home in Philadelphia and my school in Boston. The most frustrating part of the trip was a poorly designed stretch of road in and around Hartford, Connecticut, a real bottleneck that was invariably jammed with traffic. The Connecticut Highway Department had posted annoying signs at frequent intervals that made getting through it even worse. The signs had silly cartoons and cutely worded warnings to drivers that made me loathe the Connecticut Highway Department. The one that stands out in my memory was "Put Your Elbow Out Too Far — It May Go Home in Another Car!"

What business was it of the State of Connecticut whether I chose to rest my elbow on the windowsill of my car? Whoever heard of someone losing an elbow as a result of doing so? Whenever I saw that sign — and it kept popping up — I not only put my elbow out the window as far as I could but thought of putting my legs out as well and maybe my whole torso while I drove, not to mention speeding, drinking, and engaging in every other behavior that Connecticut officials didn't like.

That is roughly the effect that health promotion will have if it comes across as the finger-wagging authoritarianism of a nanny state — telling people what to do and what not to do because we think it's good for them.

Americans may be more culturally prone than others to react negatively to this kind of persuasion. A recent survey in the United Kingdom found that most people there favored greater government control of diet and public smoking. Those from higher socioeconomic groups wanted action on smoking and alcohol, while their poorer counterparts wanted good foods to be cheaper, particularly fruits and vegetables. Most people wanted the government to limit salt, fat, and sugar in foods, to ban advertising of junk foods to children, to improve school meals, and to require food labels that give nutritional values. Nine out of ten of those questioned also said that individuals should be responsible for their own health.

TAKING BACK OUR HEALTH

Individuals *should* take responsibility for their own health. But how are they going to do so unless they understand the meaning of health, know how lifestyle factors impact it, and are supported in making better choices? Certainly it is in the state's interest to encourage greater self-responsibility, but encouragement is not enough. The government has obligations to its citizens. Here are three that I consider most important:

1. Government must raise the level of health literacy in society. That will require gathering and disseminating good information and making effective education about health a national priority.
2. Government must work to make the environment more supportive of health.
3. Government must influence people's lifestyle choices — not just by telling them what they should or shouldn't do but by providing incentives for them to make good choices and disincentives to make bad ones.

At present we do not do a very good job of making people aware of the nature and importance of health and the factors that influence it. If you do an Internet search on "health promotion" or "health literacy," you will find many relevant sites, most of them governmental, but their concerns strike me as narrow and off-center. One site reports the disappointing results of a survey of American health literacy:

- 42 percent of patients could not understand directions for taking medication on an empty stomach.
- 26 percent were unable to understand the information on an appointment slip.
- 43 percent did not understand the section of a medical application that concerned their rights and responsibilities.
- 60 percent did not understand a standard informed consent.

These numbers are disappointing indeed, but they have to do with *medical* literacy, not *health* literacy. If Americans had better working knowledge of health, fewer of them would need to take medication, whether on a full or empty stomach, or need to give informed consent for procedures.

Our National Institutes of Health (NIH), a vast complex in Bethesda, Maryland, provides $28 billion annually for medical research, but little of this money brings in the kinds of information we need to meet the challenge of raising health literacy. The institutes that make up NIH are named for diseases and body parts. There is the National Cancer Institute (NCI), the National Heart, Lung, and Blood Institute (NHLBI), the National Institute of Diabetes, Digestive, and Kidney Diseases (NIDDKD), and so forth. Where is the National Institute of Health and Healing (NIHH), which ought to be at the center of the show? *It doesn't exist.*

If it did exist and I were allocating its research budget, I would put a large percentage of it into investigations of the human body's healing system and the mechanisms by which it maintains homeostasis, defends itself from harm, regenerates damaged tissue, and adapts to injury and loss. Most people do not know that the body even *has* a healing system.

I find it easier to talk about the body's healing system with children than with medical colleagues. It is very easy to implant this concept in the minds of young people by directing their attention to the repair of ordinary cuts and abrasions. The fact is that the body knows when it has been injured, and it can repair itself. If you treat it well, it will be able to do that as long as you live. Medical colleagues tend to dismiss talk of a "healing system" as New Age nonsense. It isn't. It is basic biology, and we need to make it a priority of health research and education.

OUR INNATE ABILITY TO HEAL

One of the consequences of general unawareness of the body's healing system is that too many people lack confidence in their own innate abilities to deal with common health problems. Instead of relying on the wisdom of their bodies, they seek the attention of health-care professionals and vastly overuse medical services. One way we can lower health-care costs is to teach people to be more self-reliant by increasing understanding of and confidence in their inborn capacity for healing.

Very often I have to tell patients forcefully and with all my authority as a physician that they *can* get better, that their bodies can repair themselves and recover from disease or injury. I received a call recently from a woman struggling with celiac disease, which is caused by sensitivity to gluten, the protein in wheat and other grains. Like many others with this problem, she had been misdiagnosed and improperly treated for some time, because the doctors she had seen did not recognize the pattern in her diverse symptoms (systemic, digestive, and psychological) and did not test her for gluten sensitivity. Once she had eliminated that protein from her diet, she experienced marked improvement but was still haunted by the fear that her digestive system had suffered permanent damage as a result of her delay in making the change. No one had told her, and she did not know, about the great regenerative capacity of the gastrointestinal tract. I told her that if she gave her digestive system a chance and treated it well, it could heal completely, even from extensive injury. This relieved her anxiety and speeded her recovery.

It is a no-brainer that investigating the potentials and the mechanisms of regeneration and self-healing should be a major focus of medical research. Another should be the study of disease remission. (I would direct the new National Institute of Health and Healing to make that a priority.) We do not really understand why serious chronic diseases sometimes resolve completely, either spontaneously or in response to treatment. If we knew more about the phenomenon, we might be able to make it happen more frequently. Imagine that the NIHH maintained a national registry of remission, a computerized database available to all that enabled you to locate documented case reports of remission of any disease. These records would include information about interventions that might have played a role, from conventional treatments to unorthodox ones. Furthermore, NIHH could put you or your physician in contact with people who had experienced remission of your disease and were willing to talk to you about what they had learned.

Say you were just diagnosed with multiple sclerosis, an autoimmune neurological disease that affects young adults. It can take many forms and can be disabling. It is not curable by conventional medicine but sometimes stabilizes, remits, or disappears completely. Before you took on a gloomy outlook for your future, wouldn't you like to learn about, talk to, and meet people like you who had recovered fully from MS or experienced only minimal impairment from it? Wouldn't you be delighted to know that an agency of your federal government could help you do so?

I would also expect that NIHH would be the coordinating center for research on placebo effects, long misunderstood and undervalued in our culture. Placebo effects are pure healing responses activated by mind-mediated mechanisms. Although commonly dismissed as trivial or even unreal, recent imaging studies have shown that placebo effects have a very real basis in the activity of specific areas of the brain. Just one example of a great many comes from a recent study of prostate enlargement; in this study more than half of all men who received a placebo for the condition reported significant relief, theoretically because it allowed them to relax muscles in the area of the prostate and bladder, improving urinary function.

When I speak to doctors about health and healing, I always stress the importance of placebo responses. Rather than trying to rule them out or separate them from the "real effects" of drugs and other interventions, we should try to make them happen more frequently. One way to do that is to present treatments to patients with genuine conviction of their efficacy. In integrative medicine the goal of treatment is to elicit the maximum healing response with the least invasive intervention. That approach lowers both the potential harm of treatment and its cost. To achieve it we need much better understanding of how placebos can produce real cures of even serious conditions.

Collecting this kind of information about the body's ability to maintain equilibrium and repair itself is the first half of the challenge of raising health literacy in our society. We can meet it by prioritizing relevant research, funding it generously, and centralizing the effort within a new high-profile institute in the NIH complex. The second half of the challenge is to get the information into medical education as well as the education of allied health professionals and that of the public, especially children.

Health education of the future *cannot* bear any resemblance to what I experienced in grades K-12 or to what most students still experience. In order to make Americans health literate, as a prerequisite for getting them to take greater control of their lives, education will have to be creative and highly innovative.

We have many new tools available to us, including computers, multimedia, and interactive video games that open possibilities much more exciting than those of lectures, books, and instructional films. Let me give you a few ideas I have about using video games to make young people more knowledgeable about the nature and importance of health and the profound consequences of lifestyle choices.

We tend to think of video games as one of the worst influences on young people, because they increase sedentary behavior and because many of them are graphically violent. But their positive potential is great. In a book published in 1997 titled *Health Promotion and Interactive Technology,* media consultant Debra A. Lieberman wrote, "To engage young people in health-related behaviors while they play, video games can present appealing role model characters, provide scenarios that involve making health decisions, carry out self-care skills, and depict realistic consequences in response to players' decisions and actions." That was written before the advent of immensely popular new-generation games like The Sims in which players control the actions of simulated people in a suburban household and watch them succeed or fail as the result of their decisions, or Spore, where players can create a new species of life and direct its evolution in ways that succeed in order to become more complex, powerful forms, or fail and go extinct.

Such simulation games can dramatically illustrate the consequences of lifestyle choices on health — for example, that getting insufficient physical activity promotes weight gain, which makes it harder to get dates and jobs, or that eating processed foods increases inflammation in the body along with disease risks and medical expenses (not to mention making the skin less attractive), or that practicing simple relaxation techniques can improve mood, sleep, and grades in school. Some simulation games have whole economies with virtual currencies that can be earned, saved, lost, or even exchanged for real-world goods and services, providing additional motivation to make better life decisions. Video games can also be linked to a player's real-world behavior so that his or her physical activity can be measured or daily food intake evaluated. Some use biofeedback techniques to teach stress reduction by monitoring breathing, heart rate, and skin temperature. To advance in the game you have to move those indicators in the right direction by calming the involuntary nervous system, a very useful skill. The game is self-reinforcing and provides a learning environment as far removed as possible from the "do this, don't do that" kind of instruction I got in the health classes of public schools.

These are just hints of what will be possible as game technology improves and developers put their minds to better ways of using it. The Robert Wood Johnson Foundation, the country's largest philanthropic group devoted exclusively to health and health care, has now added video game development to its "pioneer portfolio" of projects and recently cosponsored a competition for best new designs. Currently available games that are specifically designed to promote health include Ben's Game (for kids with cancer), Immune Attack, Human-Sim (focused on medical education), Medical Cyberworlds (for training physicians), Play2Train (for training first responders), and even Virtual Knee Surgery.

I believe the power of this technology to revolutionize health education and boost the health literacy of our population is formidable. I want to see it play a major role in promoting health in America.

THE GOVERNMENT'S ROLE

The federal government's public health responsibilities include health promotion. Preventive medicine deals with the health of individuals; public health deals with that of groups, societies, and populations. Many American institutions of higher learning offer programs leading to degrees in public health, and many of our academic health centers have schools of public health along with schools of medicine, nursing, pharmacy, or dentistry. The American Public Health Association (APHA) boasts that it is "the oldest and most diverse organization of public health professionals in the world and has been working to improve public health since 1872." It has about thirty thousand members.

Our national government implements policy in this area through the Department of Health and Human Services, which is responsible for protecting the health of all Americans. Its primary division is the U.S. Public Health Service, which includes the Commissioned Corps, one of our uniformed services, headed by the Surgeon General. The Department of Health and Human Services is relatively new, but the Public Health Service traces its origins to the beginnings of the country. Of the agencies within it, the one most relevant to this discussion is the Centers for Disease Control (CDC), created in 1946 with headquarters in Atlanta, Georgia. The CDC's mission is "to promote health and quality of life by preventing and controlling disease, injury, and disability," and its goals, listed prominently on its Web site, are to have

- healthy people in every stage of life.

- healthy people in healthy places.
- people prepared for emerging health threats.
- healthy people in a healthy world.

To enable the CDC to fulfill its mission and achieve these goals, Congress annually reviews the Centers' budgetary requests and appropriates funds; in fiscal year 2006 it gave the CDC a total of $8.6 billion.

Something must be wrong.

With such a well-funded and active enterprise of public health in our country one would not expect the poor health outcomes we experience compared to those of other developed countries. Far too few Americans are healthy in every stage of their lives, and far too many of them live in unhealthy places. Epidemic obesity and type-2 diabetes are two of our greatest emerging health threats, but I don't see much preparation for them. And as a chief contributor to atmospheric carbon load, America is certainly not helping to create a healthy world for its own people or any other.

Should we blame our institutions and policies of public health for these failures? Yes. As with preventive medicine, the problem is ineffective action that derives from concepts that no longer serve us. I have said that health promotion (along with disease prevention) must be a main thrust of a new system of health care. The American public health profession and the government-funded agencies that implement public health policy have to lead this effort. As they now function, they cannot do so.

A main reason is that they have their priorities wrong. In July 2008 former CDC director Julie Gerberding announced the launch of a Healthiest Nation Campaign. (Remember, America is far from being the healthiest nation.) She said, "We put way too much emphasis on treating disease, rather than protecting health in the first place," adding that "many countries have put more emphasis on health promotion" than we do. We need to focus, she continued, on the "things we need to do before we get to the doctor's office," such as building additional lanes for bicyclists and walking paths for pedestrians, offering more nutritious meal options in schools, and creating a ban on public smoking.

I couldn't agree more with Dr. Gerberding. But a look at the CDC's allocation of funds shows her words to be more lip service than commitment to action. Of the $8.4 billion the CDC received in 2006, the budget for its entire health promotion effort was a little under $1 billion. More than 30 percent of this went to cancer prevention/control, another 10 percent to tobacco-related issues. The subcategory called Nutrition, Physical Activity, and Obesity got all of $41 million — less than one-half of 1 percent of the whole 2006 budget. The best funded areas were Vaccines for Children (just under $2 billion), Infectious Diseases (slightly under $1.7 billion), and Terrorism ($1.6 billion). In other words, we spent forty times more on the health risks of terrorism than on the health risks of obesity, which kills about four hundred thousand people every year — a truly terrifying reality.

When the American Public Health Association was formed in 1872, infectious diseases were the major threat to public health. It is understandable that over the years the American enterprise of public health has directed most of its resources and activity toward improved sanitation, disinfection of public water supplies, immunization, and so forth. But now, although lifestyle-related chronic disease is far and away the greatest threat, those priorities have not changed. In fact, they have been reinforced by new fears — of bioterrorism and an influenza pandemic — as the breakdown of the CDC's budget clearly shows. The priorities *must* change if the CDC and its sister agencies are to take the lead in making health promotion the focus of the new system I envision.

If our biggest challenges are to improve outcomes and reduce cost — and they are — then we will make great inroads by, first, reducing the need to spend so much on the management of established disease. That requires more effective prevention and more effective health promotion, because a great deal of the disease we have to manage is lifestyle related. Its incidence and severity could be contained by attending to factors we can control. How can our society motivate, encourage, and, if necessary, force people to take better control of their own health and make choices that protect and maintain it rather than undermine it? We need good answers to that question before we spend any more money in the name of public health.

You may recall that prevention has two components: accurate foreseeing of danger and taking appropriate action to avoid it. I am encouraged that research on the causes of disease, including lifestyle factors, is expanding as a result of increased government funding. We know quite a bit about controllable factors that influence risks of chronic diseases, but we need to know more.

Unfortunately, that information is underemphasized in the education and training of our health professionals. A strong recommendation from a doctor — to stop smoking, for example — can more effectively motivate a patient to change harmful habits than any number of public service announcements. But doctors need to be informed and trained to present information to patients successfully (by developing proficiency in motivational interviewing, for instance). Also, as I wrote in the previous chapter, too many American physicians are misinformed about ways to reduce disease risks. Too many believe that prescribing a statin is better than addressing lifestyle issues. Why? Because their education has biased them toward pharmacological interventions and because the drug companies have undue influence on them. It would be relatively easy to change that. I will tell you how in the final chapter.

LINKING ENVIRONMENTAL HEALTH AND PERSONAL HEALTH

Another vital governmental obligation is protection and improvement of the environment, so that it supports rather than obstructs individuals from taking more responsibility for their well-being. I am sorry to say that our government has done a poor job of this. It has failed to enact and enforce sufficient measures to improve the quality of the air we breathe, the water we drink, and the soil in which we grow our food. When faced with the choice of protecting the profits of special interests or the health of the public, too often it sides with the special interests. This has become much worse in recent years with the appointments of industry bureaucrats to top positions in governmental agencies. In the past, *scientists* headed the Department of Agriculture agencies in charge of nutritional standards, agrichemical usage, food safety, and animal feedlot waste disposal. Today the directors are more likely to be corporate executives with no scientific expertise.

Perhaps the greatest environmental threat today is climate change. It will affect human health in many ways and is sure to compound our health-care woes. Many experts tell us that a warmer world will be a sicker world and that we are already in it. Certainly, we will see new infectious diseases in our population as the insect and animal vectors that carry them extend their ranges into higher latitudes, but that is just a bit of what we can expect.

The United States is the world's second largest producer of the greenhouse gases that account for the human-caused component of global warming. It is also the only developed nation that has not signed the Kyoto Protocol, the international accord that obligates signatory nations — there are now 140 of them — to reduce those emissions to significantly lower target levels by 2012. The reason? The majority of our elected officials feel that signing it would be bad for American business. In the debates in Washington about this issue, no one pointed out that the increased costs of health care resulting from human-caused climate change will be even worse for American business.

The FDA has also become unduly allied with industries that harm environmental and personal health. In August 2008 the FDA aligned itself with the chemical industry in declaring the safety of bisphenol-A (BPA), a compound used in plastic products that has been linked to hormonal disruption, developmental defects, and, most recently, increased risks of heart disease and diabetes. BPA is present to at least some degree in the bodies of an estimated 93 percent of Americans. Of particular concern is leaching of the chemical from plastic baby bottles when they are heated. Even if the toxicity of BPA is low, babies are at greater risk because of their low body weight and greater sensitivity to toxins. Although manufacturers were starting to remove bisphenol-A from products in response to consumer fears, the FDA now says it is okay even for babies.

The tendency of governments to put the short-term interests of business above long-term interests of public health is not unique to our country or our time, but it is particularly strong and harmful here and now. The nations of Europe do much better perhaps because their governments pay for nationalized health care and therefore are more invested in keeping people well.

I am also disappointed by the complacency of our citizens compared to Europeans concerning environmental issues. Americans seem not to be very bothered about — or even aware of — genetically modified (GMO) foods, while consumers in Europe successfully fought corporate efforts to force or sneak them into the market. We also allow dairy farmers to use recombinant bovine growth hormone (rBGH), an unnatural method of increasing milk production that may undermine the health of both cows and humans. Canadians were up in arms about it from the get-go and managed to ban the practice in their country.

Much of this comes down once again to our citizens' lack of knowledge, a problem that can be solved only by raising awareness through effective informational initiatives. I would hope raised awareness would lead to grassroots political movements that will help elect representatives dedicated to protecting our public health when business interests and environmental quality are at odds. The public health and medical professions *must* take the lead in collecting and disseminating the necessary information.

One of the branches of NIH is the National Institute of Environmental Health Sciences (NIEHS), whose mission is to coordinate research in this field. It has funded many studies, most of them too narrow and technical to be useful to us. But the findings of some of them are very relevant and should be better known, such as the discovery in 2002 that exposure to high concentrations of tiny particles of soot and dust from cars, power plants, and factories can raise the risk of dying from lung cancer and heart disease as much as prolonged exposure to secondhand tobacco smoke. Another finding is that children exposed to relatively small amounts of poly-chlorinated biphenyls (PCBs) before birth tend to have lower IQ scores, poorer reading comprehension, and more memory problems than other children.

We have a lot of data on environmental influences on health. We need more. And, again, we *must* get this information out there, both to health-care professionals and the general public. My medical education included nothing on this topic. Let me repeat that: *nothing.* That deficiency has not been remedied in conventional medical education to this day. However, my colleagues and I at the Arizona Center for Integrative Medicine are working to correct it by developing a curriculum in environmental health and medicine that we hope will become a required part of the training of all physicians and nurses. My passion for this project comes from my sense of how important it is to raise the environmental awareness of health-care professionals so that they can do the same for the whole society.

Doctors do not know enough at present to answer our pressing questions about the risks of cell phones, plastic water bottles, and agrichemicals. They do not know enough to be politically active and to mobilize the health-care community to counter-act the influence of corporate lobbying on environmental legislation. They do not know enough to care that our hospitals and medical centers are some of the worst pol-luters in our country, generating an average of 40 tons of solid, often toxic waste per hospital each year, or that hospitals' internal environments are inimical to health and healing. Closing this knowledge gap is an urgent priority. Only then will the health-care community be able to raise awareness of environmental influences on health and inspire action, just as it made people aware of the health consequences of smoking and laid the foundation for the antismoking movement.

In the meantime I will continue to expect our governments — national, state, and lo-cal — to fulfill their obligations in this area. Protecting the environment is integral to preventive medicine, public health, and health promotion. Correct governmental ac-tion — whether it be initiatives to limit carbon emissions by industries or better oversight by the Environmental Protection Agency (EPA) and the FDA on toxic chemi-cals — can support individuals in their ef-forts to reduce disease risks and become less dependent on the health-care system.

THE CARROT AND THE STICK

Government must also create incentives and disincentives to move people toward making better choices about how they live. That means making it easier and more rewarding for people to develop better habits of eating and physical activity, while making it harder for people to smoke by making tobacco products more expensive and less available. We have not done this in any consistent or thoughtful way. We often fail to motivate people to adopt healthier habits and even make it *easier* for them *not* to. The incentive structure of American society with regard to behavior and health is haphazard, unplanned, and rife with contradictions. Other countries do better. Germany, for one, is starting a $47 million program to encourage healthy eating, including improvements in school lunches, and is urging makers of unhealthy foods to curtail marketing to children, in part because studies indicate that banning fast-food advertising to children could reduce the number of overweight kids by as much as 18 percent.

We want people to be more physically active, but many of our cities are far from pedestrian friendly. The bicycle culture that is prominent in Scandinavia, Japan, and many other countries is overwhelmed here by our extreme car culture. Many Americans who might wish to cycle are deterred by the lack of bike lanes and the dangers of traffic. We say we want kids to be more active, but our budget priorities belie our words: Many public schools have dropped classes in physical education because of lack of funding. And we have promoted a television and Internet culture in which kids and adults are more sedentary than ever. An estimated 14 percent of our young people get no regular exercise at all, and approximately half of all people aged twelve to twenty-one are not vigorously active on a regular basis.

We want people to improve their eating habits, but we have made the unhealthiest food cheap and widely available while the most healthful foods are neither available nor affordable for many people. By underfunding public education we have forced our schools to make pacts with the devil — allowing fast-food outlets and junk food vendors onto their premises in exchange for money. Medical experts and educators wring their hands over the epidemic of childhood obesity and the rising incidence of type-2 diabetes in the very young but allow the very foods responsible for these conditions to be served in their own facilities.

What options do we have for creating a more consistent set of incentives and disincentives?

- We can use financial incentives, such as subsidies for growing fruits and vegetables, and disincentives, such as sin taxes on junk foods. We could provide tax breaks to people who maintain normal weight and exercise regularly, just as insurance companies give nonsmokers better rates. We could increase funds to schools that kick the fast-food restaurants out, provide healthy lunches, and give even more to those that offer good physical education and training in stress reduction and relaxation.

- We can also get serious about financial disincentives. In July 2008 the State of Alabama announced that overweight state employees who don't try to lose weight will have to pay part of their own health insurance premiums. They have until 2010 to start getting fit, or they will pay $25 a month for insurance that is otherwise free. Other states now reward employees who adopt health-supportive habits, but Alabama, with one of the highest rates of obesity in the country, is the first to penalize them. It already charges workers who smoke. We need to find out if these strategies work and determine the relative effectiveness of financial incentives versus disincentives.

- We can also use laws. We already have legal restrictions on sales of tobacco and alcohol. We could try legal restrictions on the advertising and marketing of foods that undermine health. We could make federal funds to states and cities contingent on their providing adequate pedestrian walkways and bike lanes or on reducing their rates of obesity. This is not a new idea. For years states have received — or not received — a portion of federal funds based on their enforcement of various driving laws, such as seat belt use.

- We can try to make unhealthy ways of living unfashionable, just as we have in part made smoking unfashionable. I have traveled in areas of our country where obesity is so common that people think it's normal. If your parents, friends, and neighbors are all overweight, why would you care if you were? Media and informational campaigns about smoking were effective counterweights to the cigarette ads that glamorized smoking. We should come up with comparable strategies for building a cultural consensus about weight management and other healthy ways of living.

As I've said, no single lifestyle is exactly right for everyone, nor do I want everyone to live the way I do. That would make for a very uninteresting society. But based on good evidence, we can offer the public general recommendations about the fundamental elements of health: diet, physical activity, drug use (including alcohol, tobacco, and caffeine), and stress; the need for adequate rest, sleep, and play; the value of social and intellectual connectedness; and the wise use of preventive medical services. We do not have to come off as lifestyle fascists or nanny-staters to motivate Americans to follow these recommendations. Our best strategy would be to help people understand *why* they should make these choices. This again is a challenge and an opportunity for educators, physicians, and government officials.

WHAT TO DO

Let me give one example of what we should be doing. Evidence is strong for the need for omega-3 fatty acids in fetal development. The fetal brain, especially in the last trimester of pregnancy, needs one of them — docosahexaenoic acid (DHA) — for optimal growth; it is a major constituent of nerve cell membranes. It is so important that when premature babies are given omega-3 fatty acids in the first few days after birth, they achieve notably higher scores on cognitive tests by the time they become toddlers. Most Americans do not get enough of these essential fats even though they're necessary for lifelong physical and mental health. In fact, our low intake may be the most serious deficiency of the mainstream diet. This is not surprising since few foods provide them. Oily fish such as salmon, sardines, and herring are the best sources, but fish consumption is low in our population and has declined even more in response to recent concerns about such toxic contaminants as mercury and polychlorinated biphenyls (PCBs).

Deficiency of DHA in pregnancy results in weakened brain structure that may predispose a child to neurological, mental, and emotional problems, from autism and

ADHD to impaired learning ability and, in later life, depression and bipolar disorder. If the mother is not consuming enough omega-3s, the fetus will rob her body and brain of DHA to try to meet its own needs, which may be the cause of postpartum depression.

What expectant mother would not want to give her baby the best chance for optimum brain health, intellectual brightness, and good resistance to emotional problems? The remedy is so simple: Supplement the diet with 2 to 3 grams of fish oil daily. (Most products are distilled to remove mercury and other contaminants.) All we have to do is *get the information out there* in the right way. Maybe we should also give fish oil capsules to women who can't afford them or reimburse them for the cost. The amount we would save in health-care expenses for conditions resulting from DHA-deficient brains would be vastly greater than the cost of doing so.

I am sure that if we as a society put our heads together, we can come up with many ways to promote better health in our country. We need to give people the information they require about the rationale for our lifestyle recommendations. And we need to make these lifestyle choices easier, cheaper, and more rewarding. We could begin with these actions:

- Create think tanks on these issues. I would like to see the big foundations interested in health care start the process. It would bring them more return on their investment than anything they have done to date.
- Direct the U.S. Department of Health and Human Services to create a new Office of Health Promotion, with funding equal to the importance of its mission. In addition to overseeing national policy, the office could coordinate state and local health promotion efforts.
- Direct the U.S. Department of Education to create its own Office of Health Education to develop innovative, effective curriculum and methods of teaching for grades K-12 and beyond. This initiative must be supported by federal funding of public school health education, including physical education.
- Direct the American Association of Medical Colleges to include information about health, healing, and health promotion in the medical school curriculum, and direct other organizations to do the same for schools of allied

health professions. (If the National Board of Medical Examiners were to include questions on these subjects in the examinations that medical students must pass, schools would quickly add them to the curriculum.)

- Organize the health-care community to counteract the power of corporate lobbies that now shape the Farm Bill, environmental legislation, and regulation of industry by the FDA, USDA, and other federal agencies. Our representatives must be made aware of the increased health-care costs resulting from present policies.

- And, of course, direct the NIH to add the National Institute of Health and Healing to its campus and allocate funds to it commensurate with its central importance in a new system, one that focuses on health promotion rather than disease management.

These actions would improve American health to a degree that is hard to imagine. They would enable the new integrative medical system of America to once again make American health care the best in the world.

CHAPTER 10
WHAT THE FUTURE
WILL LOOK LIKE

When you have a medical issue, you will come to a warm, friendly clinic or office where people know you personally and have a computerized history of your health. You will have learned the basics about your problem from information that your doctor has previously sent you and from your own Internet research. Your doctor will greet you by name, take time to find out what's happening in your life that has led to your current problem, outline an individualized, comprehensive program to help you get better (with a printout to take home), and recommend effective natural remedies and therapies unless your condition demands stronger interventions. (If it does, your doctor might refer you to a high-tech medical center or to a specialist.) You won't pay on the way out, because your doctor will bill a national plan. You will have paid for that plan, in part, with your taxes, which may be a little higher — but the thousand dollars a month you once spent on insurance will now be part of your take-home pay.

This visit will probably be a form of managed care. When opponents of nationalized health care disparage the systems in Canada and Europe, they often make "rationed care" a chief bugaboo. A professor of medicine at the University of California, Davis, wrote recently, "Any talk of rationing health care puts people on edge. In hospitals, we no longer use the word 'rationing.' Instead we discuss 'allocating scarce resources.' " Currently, most people are concerned about two questions: Who will *do* the rationing? (Excuse me: the "allocating.") And who will *get* the rations? In other words, who will be the winners and who will be the losers as health-care resources dwindle?

That is not a useful way to think. In the future, most people will understand that the depressed patient who gets better by supplementing her diet with fish oil and starting an exercise program is the winner, while the one who immediately starts long-term treatment with Zoloft is the potential loser. Similarly, the patient with coronary artery disease who improves his heart health through lifestyle modification and medication will *not* be a loser for avoiding angioplasty. Rationing of care is inevitable. One of the educational challenges of an expanded public health effort is to help people understand when they are better off *without* the most expensive interventions.

A larger question than who will do the rationing is who will do the *triaging.* "Triage," from the French verb meaning to sift, sort, or select, is the term used in conventional medicine for prioritizing patients for care (particularly the victims of mass casualty). This means separating out the deceased, who are beyond help, and then identifying those who need help immediately, those who need help but can wait, and those who are in the least need of urgent care. After the transformation of American health care, triaging will mean separating those patients who should go straight to specialized high-tech medicine from those who go to regular medicine (no longer called "integrative"). A middle-aged man with acute chest pain obviously goes right to emergency care to see if he is having a heart attack and, if so, gets appropriate medical or surgical intervention. A middle-aged man with recurrent low-back pain does not need to go a high-tech medical center.

What about patients with complaints that

may or may not indicate serious disease — a woman with abdominal pain and bloating that, however unlikely, may be symptoms of ovarian cancer, or a man with a persistent cough that is probably allergic but could come from a more dire respiratory problem? Good medical practice would include doing appropriate tests to rule out the threatening possibilities: an ultrasound examination and blood work for the woman, a chest X-ray, sputum examination, and blood work for the man. If serious disease is detected, it may be in an early stage, which is more easily treated and has a greater likelihood of cure. All patients with nonemergent conditions, including ordinary problems and chronic complaints, can be evaluated by good diagnosticians — internists, family physicians, and even general practitioners. They will sort out those who need to go to centers of high-tech medicine for diagnosis or treatment. Only this sort of triage can ensure the viability of our new system of health care, because it is the single most effective way we can target high-tech medicine to those who really need it and thereby contain medical costs.

As technology-based intervention becomes a specialty practiced in large centralized hospitals, opportunities will appear for new kinds of facilities. There will be the low-tech, low-cost doctors' offices and clinics that were once the backbone of American medicine and can be again. There will also be new, larger facilities to replace the vanished community hospitals and rural health centers. Many of these will be the kind of institution I would like to work in, one dedicated to promoting health and fostering healing, a hybrid of a clinic and a spa. Today's spas are most often "pamper resorts" that cater to the affluent, focusing on relaxation, physical fitness, and appearance. But some offer preventive medical assessments, lifestyle counseling, mind/body therapies, and other wellness services, along with the usual hikes, aerobics classes, massages, and herbal body wraps. Throughout history and in many cultures spas have been centers of health promotion and natural healing, available to both rich and poor; they are often located near hot springs. ("Spa" comes from the name of a town in Belgium that has a therapeutic spring.) In some cultures soldiers and workers were sent to spas at government expense to keep them happy and healthy, a tradition still alive in the Russian Federation and some countries of Eastern Europe.

THE HEALING CENTER

Imagine that you could go for a week to a Health and Healing Center paid for by your health insurance plan. The place would not be as opulent as a luxury spa, and the clients would be seeking health, not pampering. But it would be more than comfortable, and every aspect of it, from interior design to food, would be supportive of well-being. The center would serve people in good health as well as those with the ordinary kinds of problems that account for most doctor visits. It would be a setting for serious work on the lifestyle issues that now cause most of the chronic illness in America and that account for the near bankruptcy of the current medical system. It would not be a place for critically or terminally ill people or others who would be better served in hospitals.

Let's imagine that there is a Shenandoah Health and Healing Center in the Blue Ridge Mountains of Virginia, a facility with accommodations for two hundred guests. You are going to spend five nights there. You check in at the end of the afternoon, use the spa facilities before dinner (to exercise or relax), and then attend a group orientation and a talk about the importance of health and the body's healing system. The next morning, after breakfast and a nature walk, you meet with a health professional to review your personal medical history and plan your stay, in order to get the most out of it.

If, like most of us, you need help with eating habits, you might be advised to attend group classes on nutrition, as well as food preparation workshops, or to take a field trip to a nearby supermarket to learn how to be a health-smart shopper. You would be welcome to spend time in the kitchen's garden and greenhouse to learn about growing your own food. If, like most people, you need help with managing stress, you can choose from classes in yoga, meditation, or breath work. If you need more help, the professional who does your assessment will send you for an individual session with the resident hypnotherapist or biofeedback therapist. All guests are assessed for physical fitness and get the advice of trainers and other experts about setting realistic goals for exercise. You can try any number of activities while in residence and learn how to pursue others. You will be instructed in strategies to continue these lifestyle measures when you return to your home and work.

The Center's staff includes a sleep and

dream specialist who can help you improve your habits of rest and sleep. Besides getting practical instruction in healthy living, you would have plenty of opportunities for recreation, creative expression, and play during the week. Many guests enjoy the laughter therapy groups, for example, where they experience the health-promoting effects of that behavior. You would be inspired by the staff. Everyone who works at the Center, from receptionists to therapists to waiters in the dining room, exemplifies healthy living.

Transformed medicine will depend on the collaborative efforts of practitioners from various healing traditions, under the direction of generalists with an integrative perspective. The Center's professional staff includes naturopathic and osteopathic physicians, body workers and mind/body therapists, psychotherapists, Chinese medicine practitioners, and more. Their services will be used selectively where they are most cost-effective. For instance, if you suffer from ulcerative colitis, you might be sent to Chinese medicine. If chronic back pain is a problem, you might go to a mind/body practitioner or to therapeutic yoga. The overall goal would be to help you learn how to manage these problems on your own and be less dependent on medication and professional services, both conventional and unconventional.

By the time these health and healing centers are operative, we will have ample data from large outcomes studies to justify paying people to use them. I am quite confident that the data will document the profound benefits of such facilities, both in better health and reduced costs.

An initial weeklong stay with shorter annual visits for lifestyle tune-ups will be sound investments in public health. The costs will pale in comparison to those of conventional crisis management medicine, such as the half-million dollars that cancer treatment often requires or the thousands of dollars that is spent on treatment every year for every person with heart disease.

When you check out of the Shenandoah Center for Health and Healing at the end of your week, you will be refreshed and ready to get back to your daily routine. You will have had a vacation, but you will also have learned about living well. You will know more about your capacity for healing and how you can effectively maintain your health and manage minor ailments. You will understand how much of your health and well-being is really in your control. You will have greater confidence in your own ability to take care of any health problems that might arise and will know more about specific professional services that would be most helpful to you. Your stay will have empowered you to be more self-reliant and less dependent on the health-care system.

I foresee a nationwide network of these centers, available to all. At the start maybe only some insurers will reimburse for visits to them, and maybe only in part, but as we move toward a more efficient single-payer system, this should be included in our health care. Year by year we should see greater utilization of the new facilities and less traffic to the regional centers of high-tech medicine.

Smaller, simpler versions of these new spa/clinic hybrids will appear in many towns. People might visit them for as little as a few hours at a time; however they are used, they will help us achieve a most important goal: the creation of a new culture of health.

THE TRANSFORMATION TO INTEGRATIVE MEDICINE

The current system of disease management, reliant as it is on exorbitantly priced ineffective drugs, is so corrupted and so lacking in new ideas that it is now collapsing under the weight of its own failures. Sooner or later it will be replaced by an integrative system that combines the best ideas and practices of conventional medicine with an expanded range of therapies and emphasizes disease prevention and health promotion. Let's hope this happens sooner. As I've mentioned, the average health-care costs for a family of four are now about $33,000 per year, and this will double in just several years. So it is important that we all do as much as we can to speed the change before we are overwhelmed with debt and disease. There are several very basic but difficult steps we need to take.

I believe it is inevitable that America will have to provide universal access to health care. Any elected official who denounces universal health care as "socialized medicine" should be turned out of office. If a majority of voters do not share that opinion, then the challenge is to educate them. We must develop thoughtful arguments and clear explanations — for example, that an efficient national system of health care (1) will save tremendous amounts of money now wasted inexcusably in administrative costs, (2) will not compromise free choice of physicians or hospitals, and (3) will improve our dreadful health outcomes relative to those of other developed countries. I want to see teams of experts in policy, health care, economics, and communications begin to craft those arguments. Then, using the media in effective, creative ways, we have to disseminate them to build the necessary consensus.

People must also understand that freeing medicine from its present corporate trap does not mean preventing doctors from making good livings commensurate with their skill and the time they have invested in their training, nor does it mean that manufacturers of medical equipment and pharmaceutical medications should not make fair profits. What it does mean is that American health care will not continue to develop as a fiercely profit-driven industry. It also means that American medicine can flourish only in a *system that places greater value on health outcomes and the welfare of providers and patients than on bottom-line profit.*

THE NEED TO BE HEARD

Most physicians I know understand this very well. Many are bitterly angry about the circumstances in which they are forced to work, but they do not know how to channel their anger into constructive action for change. Their professional organizations could help, but most of them don't. The AMA, which now represents only a minority of American physicians (far less than one-third), is notably passive. In some areas of the country doctors have formed labor unions and have gone on strike to demand better working conditions, which is probably not a good strategy for professional caregivers. I would love to see them get more involved in politics. Chiropractors have been much more active over the years; many have even held elective office. As a result, chiropractors have succeeded in getting most of what they set their sights on: licensure in all states, the right to use X-rays, reimbursement under Medicare, and so forth. By contrast, very few medical doctors have sat in legislatures, and the medical profession has been relatively ineffective at protecting and advancing its interests.

Patients are every bit as angry as doctors with American health care. They have a lot to say, and they want to be heard. What is missing is a forum for both physicians and patients to share their distressing experiences, to express their anger, and to direct it appropriately.

What might such a forum look like? I

would love to see a major national summit meeting on health-care reform, followed by a nationwide series of town meetings. Panels of experts from various fields could coordinate the events, answer questions, and encourage people to take action. I would happily participate in meetings like this, because I believe they could start a political movement for real reform. We cannot depend on politicians to initiate such a movement. On both sides of the aisle they have proved themselves incapable of it; they are devoid of vision and unwilling to disengage from the vested interests.

In June 2004 *Time* magazine and ABC News convened a three-day national Summit on Obesity in Williamsburg, Virginia, that featured many expert speakers. It was very well attended. The Robert Wood Johnson Foundation funded the event, and because of the nature of the sponsoring organizations, it was widely publicized in print and on television and radio. The Summit on Obesity brought overdue national attention to a serious problem through the combined power of two leading news organizations and America's largest foundation dedicated to health and health care. I would ask these institutions to do it again, this time on the even tougher problems discussed in this book, such as rethinking our model of disease prevention, getting medicine up to speed with the rest of science in embracing complexity, and organizing the outcomes studies we need to change priorities of reimbursement. Then I would ask them to enroll other media and foundation partners to organize the town meetings. Agenda items might include these: how to bring prevention and health promotion to the forefront of our health-care system; how to increase the understanding of health among our citizens, including doctors and patients; how to reduce the billions of dollars of administrative waste in the present system; and how the Internet can make us healthier.

To implement the major changes in our perceptions and delivery of health care, we need a consensus of public opinion and a mobilization of public will. Those of us who realize the importance of these goals must work, individually and collectively, to raise awareness of the issues, to find ways of addressing them, and to make this part of the everyday American dialogue. Our health-care professionals should take the lead here.

Here are some possibilities:

Creating a Public Discussion
About Reform

- Medical students (and students of allied health professions) can form discussion groups on health-care reform and petition faculties and administrators for needed changes in curriculum. Medical students have successfully agitated for instruction in CAM and for access to courses such as The Healer's Art. Pharmacy students should be demanding instruction in appropriate uses of natural therapeutic agents, including botanicals, vitamins, and other dietary supplements. Nursing students should be ardent activists for reform, because underpayment of nurses is one reason for the nationwide shortage of nursing care that is a significant factor in the deterioration of American health care.

- Doctors can form action groups within their professional organizations, with the goal of making them agencies for change. The American College of Physicians (ACP) is a 126,000-strong organization of internists and internal medicine subspecialists, residents, and fellows. If it were to call for federal subsidies of residency training in pre-

ventive medicine and primary care, the
call would be taken seriously. If the
American Medical Association and
American Hospital Association were to
take strong stands against fast-food
restaurants in hospitals, things would
change.

- Other health professionals can do the
same. A few years ago I spoke to the
annual meeting of the American Di-
etetic Association, where the thousands
of registered dieticians in attendance
all carried conference tote bags advertising aspartame (NutraSweet), an
artificial sweetener that has no place in
a healthy diet. Growing numbers of
RDs understand that; it is time for
them to force their professional organization to disassociate itself from inappropriate corporate sponsorship.
- Editors of medical journals can call for
submissions of articles proposing new
models of health care. In July 2008 the
American Journal of Medicine ran an
editorial by Drs. James Dalen and Joseph Alpert proposing mandatory
national not-for-profit health insurance
financed by a payroll tax shared by employees and employers. Patients would
have free choice of physicians, other

health-care providers, and hospitals, while physicians would be paid fees for service. The authors argued that their proposed system would end the enormous administrative costs that now drag us down, end the profit-driven abuses of the insurers, and greatly improve the health of our population. "The major reason that our health outcomes are poor," they wrote, "is that more than 46 million Americans have limited access to care because they don't have health insurance." This is the kind of writing I have in mind: a clear, concise argument for a specific transformative, forward-thinking, cost-effective initiative. I'd like to see more such articles in professional publications on a range of possibilities for better delivery of health care.

- Foundations whose mission includes health and health care, perhaps in partnership with universities, can assemble think tanks of experts from different fields to tackle such questions as these: What would a national system of health care look like? What would it cost? Who will pay for it? How can we move American medicine into a not-for-profit mode? How do we develop and implement a legislative agenda to change the system?

- These groups should be directed to come up with specific, actionable proposals to be put in the hands of people with influence. (Some of the foundations that are now most forward-thinking on health-care reform are: the Robert Wood Johnson Foundation, the Henry J. Kaiser Family Foundation, Families USA, and the Center for Studying Health System Change. See the appendix of this book for information about how to contact them and other relevant organizations.)
- Corporations struggling to contain spending on health care can seek partnerships with government agencies and academic centers to evaluate the clinical effectiveness and cost-effectiveness of innovative ways of managing common health problems of workers, especially integrative treatment.
- Patients can join organized efforts to change reimbursement policies of the big insurers so that they pay equitably for preventive care, lifestyle counseling, and interventions other than drugs and surgery. As I have explained, many

of the existing alternatives to drastic treatment have low potential for harm, show reasonable evidence for efficacy, and are both time- and cost-effective.

Apart from any organizations or groups, your voice as an individual consumer of health care counts toward the consensus needed to create a new system, and if you are well informed, you can persuade people you know to be part of it. Start by learning more about the seriousness of the crisis and how it will affect you. Will you be able to pay your health insurance premiums? What are you getting in return? Are you satisfied with the quality of health-care services you have used? What would happen to you economically if you or a family member had to deal with devastating illness or injury?

A public forum and national dialogue will be a good start. But to achieve the transformation that health care requires, we also need a prolonged, nationwide, coordinated campaign of *action*. Here are the most important actions we need to take to make American health the best in the world instead of the thirty-seventh best.

- We must radically revise the *entire conversation* about health-care reform in America. Right now we're obsessed with devising new ways to save the old dysfunctional system. That won't happen, because it is fundamentally flawed, and billions of dollars more will not bail it out. Instead of throwing good money after bad, we need to put our best minds to work on implementing disease prevention, health promotion, and integrative medicine.

We need to convene conferences, seminars, task forces, and think tanks to develop strategies for prevention and promotion that are realistic and scientifically sound (and that account for complexity). Universities, foundations, and government agencies, including the CDC, should take the lead.

- It is imperative that the pharmaceutical drug industry be drastically reformed: by increased governmental oversight, by consumer boycotts and other actions of protest, and by vigorous investigation in the media. The pharmaceutical industry now dominates American medicine to a degree that was unimaginable thirty years ago, and much of what is now wrong with that industry is what is wrong with American health care: Most fundamentally it is high costs and poor results. The free market has failed us here. Tighter regulation of big pharma is long overdue and urgently needed.

We must vigorously lobby Congress for much stricter regulation of the industry. We should insist on an immediate ban of direct-to-consumer advertising of prescription drugs. We must reduce and try to eliminate the corruptive influence of pharmaceutical advertising on the content and editorial practices of medical journals. I would like to see a nonprofit foundation convene a summit of editors in chief of the leading journals to discuss ways of doing that.

The federal government must enact price controls on prescription drugs covered by Medicare, and Medicare should cover *all* effective treatments, not just pharmaceuticals. It should reimburse for appropriate dietary supplements and natural therapies — everything from multivitamins and fish oil to licorice extract (DGL) as well as therapeutic yoga and guided imagery audio programs.

Government must institute strict reviews

of all drug advertising for distorted claims of safety and efficacy, and institute much tougher standards for the approval of new drugs, particularly with regard to evidence for safety. After new drugs are introduced, they must be reviewed on a regular basis to weed out those that do not meet reasonable standards of safety or efficacy — before catastrophe strikes.

The federal government should subsidize the preparation, publication, and distribution of an *objective* standard reference source for health professionals on the uses, benefits, and risks of prescription drugs. This would replace the *Physician's Desk Reference* (PDR), an industry publication now in universal use that encourages physicians to use these products. A federal commission should be appointed to do this, drawing on academic experts and, especially, on the expertise of *The Medical Letter,* an independent, not-for-profit periodical that has been publishing relatively unbiased information about drugs since 1959 but whose readership and influence on American medicine are insignificant compared to those of the PDR. (Another excellent objective resource is *The Pharmacist's Letter,* which also makes available a useful *Natural Medicines Comprehensive Database.*) A federal agency should also create a Web site, available to everyone, that would enable consumers to evaluate for themselves the relative benefits and risks of various drugs.

To end the pharmaceutical industry's domination of information about treatment of disease, licensing agencies should require physicians, physicians' assistants, nurse practitioners, and pharmacists to be familiar with non-pharmacological interventions for the management of common health conditions, such as an anti-inflammatory diet for allergies and autoimmunity, breath work for anxiety disorders, exercise and supplemental fish oil for mild to moderate depression, etc. Schools and licensing agencies should create new proficiency exams in nutrition, lifestyle, and mind/body interventions for all providers; they should be designed to assess how well they can counsel patients.

Laws should strongly restrict drug company representatives from unethically influencing the prescribing practices of physicians through false information or any other type of deception. When there are mass deaths from drugs that are improperly tested and represented, the responsible persons should be held liable in civil and possibly even criminal proceedings.

The federal government must either abolish the Food and Drug Administration and replace it with a new agency adequately funded and purged of corporate influences, or restructure it completely. The agency should create within it a Center for Evaluation and Investigation of Natural Therapeutic Agents to study and regulate the use of vitamins, minerals, herbs, dietary supplements, and other natural products. This Center must be staffed by scientists familiar with complexity, who understand the important differences between the composition and actions of whole natural products compared to isolated chemicals. One mission of the new FDA will be to ensure the safety and quality of natural therapeutic agents on the market, not to thwart consumer access to them.

- Physicians, other health professionals, and activist citizens must begin to pressure the American Association of Medical Colleges to address deficiencies in undergraduate medical education — for example, in nutrition, mind/body interactions, lifestyle medicine, botanical medicine, CAM, etc. As I've noted, one strategy would be to lobby the National Board of Medical Examiners to include questions on these subjects in National Board exams that medical students must pass. That would immediately force medical school faculties to begin teaching them.

The president must also direct the U.S. Department of Education to support education and training in integrative medicine. A good place to start would be subsidizing the development of a comprehensive IM curriculum to be included in all medical residency training, because IM curriculum development and implementation are expensive. The executive branch should also direct the U.S. Department of Health and Human Services, perhaps through the Health Resources and Services Administration (HRSA), to do the same.

- We need to begin immediately to increase the number of generalists in medical practice. Only 11 percent of U.S. physicians engage in general practice or family practice, compared to 50 percent in Canada and 67 percent in Australia. (The Australian health-care system is in much less trouble than ours.) As I have explained, we will need generalists to triage patients in the new system of health care that I envision, sorting out the minority of those who should go to conventional medical clinics for technology-based diagnostic and therapeutic services from the majority, who can benefit more from integrative care.

The reason that specialized medicine attracts more young physicians is simply that it offers better-paying jobs (and more prestige). The corrective measure is to subsidize the training and increase the salaries of primary care doctors. I would ask HRSA to take the lead here, but it will require a directive and funds from Congress. One possibility is to forgive student loans of those who opt to become primary care providers.

- The executive branch should upgrade the National Center for Complementary and Alternative Medicine at NIH to a full-fledged institute with funding comparable to that of other major components of NIH. It should be renamed the National Institute for Integrative Medicine and can include a center for research on CAM. A function of this agency would be to develop and test models for delivery of IM services, including multidisciplinary teams of providers. These models can eventually evolve into the Health and Healing Centers that I described in this chapter.

This new agency should also test the value and cost-effectiveness of a sixty-minute initial consultation with all patients. In addition, it should be able to designate particular schools, corporations, and communities that excel in providing healthy environments, and offer them tangible rewards, including tax credits for the private sector and increased federal funding for the public sector. These entities should also be a focus of research in order to measure the value of their efforts.

- The insurance industry must be radically restructured, preferably as a nonprofit industry or as part of a single-payer entity. The industry is arguably the single most dysfunctional component of American health care, because it now meets its financial obligations to its shareholders by charging consumers as much as possible while providing as little service as possible. It can get away with this because so many people feel that they must have insurance, freeing the industry from the market forces of supply and demand that usually promote quality and fairness. And unlike other forms of insurance, health insurance is usually purchased for groups, giving individuals little power to negotiate.

Congress and the executive branch of the federal government should enact tighter controls on claim denials and should stop the insurance industry from controlling medical practice through its reimbursement policies. Congress must also put reasonable limits on price increases and should help create a transition to a system of reimbursement in which insurance profits do not reduce health resources.

Insurance companies should be compelled to reimburse for integrative medical services, including group visits. For example, lifestyle interventions and relaxation training can be done efficiently with groups of patients with hypertension or type-2 diabetes, allowing patients to benefit from group support while providers make maximum use of their time.

- The federal government should step up its effort to develop a national system of electronic medical records that are available to all patients and health-care facilities — with appropriate privacy protection. This would help reduce the billions of dollars wasted annually in administrative costs (now accounting for 31 percent of our total health-care expenses). We will also need to revise billing procedures as we move toward a single-payer system. Many of these and other initiatives that must occur to reform health care can be funded with money saved by making the present system more efficient.
- The final effort that must be made to transform our health-care system is possibly the most important of all: greater individual adherence to the principles of healthy living. To paraphrase Gandhi, we must be the change that we seek.

Really, this is more an opportunity than a burden, because it does not depend on changing the government, the insurance system, or the big corporations. However dysfunctional our present health-care system is, it is *relatively easy* for individuals to remove themselves from the disease management model and adopt the basic, simple lifestyle measures that promote optimum health: good diet, adequate physical activity and sleep, stress management, avoidance of toxins, use of natural remedies, and the limitation of pharmaceutical drugs to those situations that really require them. You may well have already begun to do all this, but if not, you can start today.

MOVING TO PREVENTION AND PROMOTION

Throughout this book I have insisted that a free democratic society must guarantee basic health care to all its citizens and that this must not be thwarted by medicine that operates in a predominantly for-profit mode, with the collusion of a rapacious insurance industry and a passive government. But today about 47 million Americans receive *no* guarantee of basic health care from a system that is hobbled by profit-driven managed care, by an insurance industry that rakes in profits, and by politicians who don't seem to care. This should make us furious, especially as we watch the economic collapse of a system we have spent billions on and once trusted with our lives.

Correcting these problems will require a massive societal effort, including legislative initiatives that our present elected representatives are unable or unwilling to support due to their subservience to special interests. If we want real change, we will have to elect new representatives, and we will have to do a lot of the work ourselves. It is up to us to muster the necessary political will.

I present here an agenda that we should all be working for. It includes laws to be passed, government policies to be refashioned, institutional reforms, improvement of professional training and practice, and more. At the end of this book I list resources that you can contact for further information, organizations you can join to work for change, and people and agencies you can call, write, or e-mail to express your support for these goals. These recommendations for action are addressed to *all* readers — citizens young and old, physicians, nurses, hospital administrators, small-business owners, legislators, the healthy and the not so healthy. They are not just for people who care about health-care reform but for everyone who cares about our nation, our economy, and our way of life.

- Our insurance companies must be

compelled, by the government and by the *buyers* of insurance, to change their priorities of reimbursement to favor prevention, health promotion, and lifestyle medicine. The day the insurers accept as reimbursable Current Procedural Terminology (CPT) codes for preventive and health-promoting services is the day doctors will begin offering them in earnest.

- Our medical schools must teach disease prevention and health promotion along with disease management and crisis intervention. Our government, medical profession, and business interests must promote and at least partially subsidize residency training in preventive medicine and public health. And they must ensure that the salaries of people entering these fields reflect their importance and are competitive with those of other specialists.

- We must create a National Institute of Health and Healing within the NIH, fund it appropriately, and give it clear directives for research initiatives. Its first order of business is to set up the National Registry of Disease Remission. Creating an institute of health and healing is not a utopian ideal but a practical necessity. We must also urge the federal government to create an Office for Health Promotion within the U.S. Department of Health and Human Services and give it sufficient funding to carry out its mission. In addition, there must be a federal mandate that at least 20 percent of the CDC's annual budget be devoted to health promotion. We cannot possibly control the present epidemic of chronic lifestyle-related disease until we learn how to promote health. Therefore, there should also be a new Office of Health Education within the U.S. Department of Education. Its mission would be to develop and implement innovative K-12 education about health, healing, and disease prevention using standard methods as well as educational tools that are especially persuasive to children, such as interactive video games. If we can create a new generation of Americans who are truly health conscious, our epidemic of chronic disease will become a historic footnote like the last century's epidemic of contagious disease.

- Citizens must pressure the American Hospital Association, the American

Public Health Association, the CDC, and other relevant governmental agencies to make the greening of our hospitals and medical centers a top priority so that the hospitals themselves don't create even more illness. Hospitals are the fourth leading source of discharge into the environment of mercury, one of the most toxic substances on earth. That's unacceptable as well as absurd. The greening of our hospital system means not only reducing their contribution to the pollution of the environment but also redesigning their internal environments to promote health and healing. A good first step would be banning sales of fast food, junk food, and other unhealthy products on their premises.

- We need to accept the seemingly obvious fact that the environment can make people sick and that no amount of medical intervention can protect us. Health-care providers must therefore broaden their intellectual and political horizons to become involved in environmental issues. They need to work to protect us from diseases that don't need to occur. We must mobilize the health-care community to become a forceful political lobby on environmental policy and legislation, federal farm policy, and other matters that directly affect the health of our people and the expense of managing preventable diseases. When mobilized, this community can neutralize the power of the corporate lobbies that now have their way with Congress and state legislatures. We must also increase funding of the National Institute of Environmental Health Sciences and give it clearer direction to focus attention on the most clinically relevant issues in environmental health.

- We need to support grassroots movements to promote health by working to ban sales of soft drinks and junk foods in public schools, getting our schools serious about physical education and health education, and fighting attempts by agribusiness to weaken federal organic standards. An aroused public can move our government's do-nothing agencies into action, and there is no shortage of health-related issues that need action, from climate change to tobacco addiction to epidemic obesity.
- As the customers of the American

media, we need to insist (with the power of our pocketbooks) that our newspapers, TV networks, and movie studios use their tremendous influence in a positive way. The media now shower us with destructive advertising, illness-promoting images (such as those of people smoking and kids devouring junk food), and shallow news reports about health and medicine that often play on our fears. We can use creative public service messages on radio, television, and the Internet to counteract the influence of harmful advertising. If these messages are delivered by celebrities, they can help make healthy living more glamorous and fashionable. We also need a new generation of investigative medical journalists who don't just parrot the party lines of conventional medicine but probe deeply enough into medical outcomes and costs to expose the deceit and hypocrisy that now pervade health care.

- Directors of small businesses and large corporations must realize that they don't need to get stuck with outrageous insurance bills for their employees every month. This doesn't happen in most other developed countries, and it is a major reason that American business is struggling. Our companies are being terribly exploited, not just by insurers but also by those elements of the disease management industry that *consume* most of the money that comes from insurance premiums: drug companies, medical device makers, highly paid specialists, and for-profit hospitals. The current economic crisis should be proof enough that American businesses cannot flourish in the global marketplace while they are being fleeced in their own country. In addition, we need to convince corporate America that it is suffering unnecessary damage from preventable employee absenteeism and diminished productivity, and that it can benefit enormously by offering workers discounted gym memberships, smoking cessation programs, and more nutritious cafeteria food. Ultimately, American corporations might even take responsibility for shaping the tastes of consumers and moving their customers in directions that are more consistent with good health.

THE BEGINNING OF THE NEW
AMERICAN MEDICINE

At this point we are not close to true health-care reform in America. Too many people — some of whom have good motives, and some of whom don't — are trying to prop up a failed system. But at least discussion of reform is finally beginning. For many years it was shunted aside by the many powerful business interests that have long profited from disease management and from sales of products that cause disease. If the current economic crisis had not hit, this discussion would probably still be blocked. But Americans have been pushed to their limits, physically and financially, and new voices are finally being heard.

Many people I know feel helpless to do anything about the crisis we face. The forces arrayed against change seem huge and implacable: heartless insurance companies, failing hospitals, greedy health-care corporations, ineffectual public servants, impersonal managed care, bureaucracy, lack of intelligible information, and, always, staggering expense. These realities seem so overwhelming that it is not surprising so many people are pessimistic. But that will change.

A Final Word

In the opening chapter of this book I promised that I would cover two big topics: (1) moving the focus of health care from disease management to prevention and health promotion, and (2) minimizing interventional medicine's dependence on expensive technology. By relying on integrative medicine to make these big changes, I am certain we will improve health outcomes and bring costs down. This is the *radix* — the root of the health-care crisis.

I have shared with you my best ideas about how to solve the crisis, and I have tried to paint pictures of what radically transformed health care might look like. Please do not dismiss these possibilities as pipe dreams or utopian fantasies. What I envision is possible and practical. As soon as we start to implement it, we will see American health improve and the cost of American health care come down.

This transformation will be one of our greatest achievements.

I invite you to join me in making it happen.

ACKNOWLEDGMENTS

I am very pleased to have a new home at Hudson Street Press and thank the editor in chief, Caroline Sutton, for making the production of this book such a streamlined and painless process.

My literary agent and friend Richard Pine recognized from the start the importance of what I was writing and got the manuscript into the right hands. I am deeply appreciative of his experience, skill, and support.

Two talented writers helped me on this project. Andrew Postman did a great deal of research for the book. By summarizing published information and interviewing experts for me, he was able to provide material I needed. Cameron Stauth helped improve the organization of the book and bolster my arguments with data. Without his assistance I could not have completed the writing on schedule.

My colleague, Victoria Maizes, M.D.,

executive director of the Arizona Center for Integrative Medicine, read various drafts of the manuscript and made valuable suggestions.

Several friends also read early drafts and gave me useful comments, among them Winifred Rosen, Dr. Jim Nicolai, and Scotty Johnson.

Finally, I thank all those colleagues, friends, and others who are working to make integrative medicine the mainstream force in health care of the future. In particular, I thank Senator Tom Harkin of Iowa for his unwavering support.

Andrew Weil
Vail, Arizona
May 2009

APPENDIX:
RESOURCES AND
INFORMATION

Books

Abramson, John. *Overdo$ed America: The Broken Promise of American Medicine.* New York: Harper Perennial, 2005.

Angell, Marcia. *The Truth About the Drug Companies: How They Deceive Us and What to Do About It.* New York: Random House, 2005.

Cohn, Jonathan. *Sick: The Untold Story of America's Health Care Crisis — and the People Who Pay the Price.* New York: HarperCollins, 2007.

Herzlinger, Regina E. *Who Killed Health Care? America's $2 Trillion Medical Problem — and the Consumer-Driven Cure.* New York: McGraw-Hill, 2007.

Quadagno, Jill. *One Nation Uninsured: Why the U.S. Has No National Health Insurance.* New York: Oxford University Press, 2005.

Relman, Arnold S. *A Second Opinion: Rescu-*

ing America's Health Care. New York: Public Affairs, 2007.

Richmond, Julius B., and Rashi Fein. *The Health Care Mess: How We Got Into It and What It Will Take to Get Out.* Cambridge, Mass.: Harvard University Press, 2005.

Starr, Paul. *The Social Transformation of American Medicine.* New York: Basic Books, 1982.

Sullivan, Kip. *The Health Care Mess: How We Got Into It and How We'll Get Out of It.* Bloomington, Ind.: AuthorHouse, 2006.

Terry, Ken. *RX for Health Care Reform.* Nashville: Vanderbilt University Press, 2007.

Web Sites

www.whyourhealthmatters.com will provide you with developing information on the issues covered in this book.

www.drweil.com will give you information to help you take greater responsibility for your health and wellness.

www.integrativemedicine.arizona.edu is the Web site of the Arizona Center for Integrative Medicine (AzCIM). You can locate practitioners the Center has trained by following the link "Find a Practitioner." AzCIM is committed to changing our health-care system. Forward-thinking philanthropists have funded many of its initiatives.

www.imconsortium.org, the Consortium of Academic Health Centers for Integrative Medicine, is a membership organization of medical schools in the United States and Canada committed to paradigm change in education, research, and clinical practice.

www.bravewell.org, the Bravewell Collaborative, is a philanthropic community working to "return healing to medicine" by advancing integrative medicine.

www.weilfoundation.org, the Weil Foundation, supports the advancement of integrative medicine through training, research, the education of the public, and policy reform.

Other Resources

Here are several helpful foundations, government agencies, advocacy groups, Web sites, and other media devoted to health-care issues:

Alliance for Health Reform (allhealth.org)
American Public Health Association (apha.org)
Center for Studying Health System Change (hschange.com)

Centers for Disease Control and Prevention (cdc.org)

Families USA (familiesusa.org)

Henry J. Kaiser Family Foundation (kff.org)

National Coalition on Health Care (nchc.org)

National Institute of Environmental Health Sciences (niehs.nih.gov)

Robert Wood Johnson Foundation (rwjf.org)

Science Daily (sciencedaily.com)

SEIU (Service Employees International Union) on Health Care (seiu.org/seiuhealthcare/index.php)

Trust for America's Health (healthyamericans.org)

U.S. Department of Health and Human Services (hhs.gov)

WebMD (webmd.com)

"Well," the *New York Times* health blog (well.blogs.nytimes.com)

NOTES

Chapter 1. You Have a Right to Good Health Care

A recent survey of U.S. primary care providers: "Overrated Careers 2009 (Physician)" by Marty Nemko, *U.S. News & World Report,* Dec. 11, 2008 (www.usnews.com); based on a survey by the Physicians Foundation.

We spend more per capita on health care than any other nation: "U.S. Health Care Spending: Comparison with Other OECD Countries" by C. Peterson and R. Burton, *Congressional Research Report for Congress* (RL34175), Sept. 2007, assets.open crs.com/rpts/RL34175_20070917.pdf.

We are at or near the bottom compared to other developed countries: "Mirror, Mirror on the Wall: An International Update on the Comparative Performance of American Health Care" by K. Davis et al., *The Commonwealth Fund,* May 15, 2007,

www.commonwealthfund.org/Content/
Publications/Fund-Reports/2007/May/
Mirror--Mirror-on-the-Wall--An-Interna
tional-Update-on-the-Comparative-Per
formance-of-American-Healt.aspx#cita
tion.

*Every thirty seconds someone in America files
for bankruptcy:* "Health Crisis: 'A Bankruptcy Every 30 Seconds' " by D. Lothian,
CNNMoney.com, Mar. 5, 2009, money
.cnn.com/2009/03/05/news/healthcare_
summit/index.htm.

*The Congressional Budget Office reports that
50 percent of recent increases:* "Technological Change and the Growth of Health
Care Spending," CBO, Jan. 2008,
www.cbo.gov/ftpdocs/89xx/doc8947/01-
31-TechHealth.pdf.

*The World Health Organization recently rated
America thirty-seventh:* "The World Health
Organization's Ranking of the World's
Health Systems," www.geographic.org,
photius.com/rankings/healthranks.html.
Also: "World's Best Medical Care?" edito-
rial, *New York Times,* Aug. 12, 2007.

**Chapter 2. Exposing the Myths of
American Health Care**

The New York Times *noted the following in
2007:* "World's Best Medical Care?" edito-

rial, *New York Times,* Aug. 12, 2007.

In a ranking of developed countries by the Centers for Disease Control and Prevention: "Infant Mortality: U.S. Ranks 29th" by Daniel J. DeNoon, *WebMD HealthNews,* Oct. 15, 2008, www.webmd.com.

In an eight-country ranking, the United States came in last: "World's Best Medical Care?" editorial, *New York Times,* Aug. 12, 2007.

The incidence of cancer has risen since 1975, not decreased: www.cancer.org/docroot/STT/STT_0.asp.

Eight percent of all Americans have diabetes: "Diabetes Statistics," American Diabetes Association, www.diabetes.org/diabetes-statistics.jsp.

The survival rates for several cancers have increased only slightly: "Long-term Survival Rates of Cancer Patients Achieved by the End of the 20th Century: A Period Analysis" by Hermann Brenner, *Lancet* 360, Oct. 12, 2002, pp. 1131–35. *Also:* "Alternative Vs. Orthodox Cancer Treatments," quoting U.S. Dept. of Commerce, www.articlesbase.com/medicine.

Survival with lung cancer: "Survival Benefit Minimal Despite Rising Cost of Lung Cancer Treatment in Elderly" by R. Nelson, *Medscape Medical News,* Oct. 25, 2007, www.medscape.com/viewarticle/

564872.

The type of brain cancer suffered by Senator Edward Kennedy: "Senator Kennedy Diagnosed with Brain Cancer," *Cancer Monthly,* May 21, 2008.

Approximately one in five Americans has arthritis: From a study by the Centers for Disease Control and Prevention for the National Arthritis Data WorkGroup, www.cdc.gov/arthritis/data_statistics/state_data.htm.

America's obesity rate is the worst in the world: www.scribd.com/doc/2415430/Countries-with-the-highest-obesity-rates. *Also:* "Germans are Fattest People in Europe, Study Shows," *Spiegel Online International,* Apr. 19, 2007, www.spiegel.de/international.

The average prescription now costs $70: Prescription Drug Trends, Kaiser Family Foundation, Sept. 2008; http://www.kff.org/rxdrugs/3057.cfm.

Cancer treatment can easily cost: www.redorbit.com/news/health/1310567/patients_dealing_with_rising_cancer_treatment_costs/.

Our health care now consumes approximately one-sixth of the American economy: "Facts on Health Care Costs," National Coalition on Health Care, www.nchc.org/

documents/cost_fact_sheet_2008.pdf. *Also:* "Getting There from Here," *The New Yorker,* Annals of Public Policy, Jan. 26, 2009, www.newyorker.com.

The U.S. medical device industry generated more than $75 billion in revenues in 2006: "Overview of the Medical Device Industry," University of California, Berkeley, www.unex.berkeley.edu.

The pharmaceutical industry dwarfs it: "Marketing Drugs: Debating the Real Cost," State Legislatures Magazine, www.ncsl.org, Sept. 2008. *Also: The Truth About Drug Companies: How They Deceive Us and What to Do About It* by Marcia Angell, Random House, New York, 2005.

The pharmaceutical industry claims that it needs high profits: "Pharmaceutical Company Profits and Salaries," data from SEC 10K filings and 1999 Company Annual Reports, www.actupny.org.

It is estimated that chronic illnesses account for 75 to 80 percent of America's total health-care bill: "Health Care That Works for All Americans," Citizens' Health Care Working Group; www.allhealth.org/BriefingMaterials/invitationtomakehealth care-221.pdf.

Recent research reported in the Journal of Clinical Investigation: "Maternal High-fat

Diet Triggers Lipotoxicity in the Fetal Livers of Nonhuman Primates" by C. McCurdy et al., *Journal of Clinical Investigation* 119(2), Feb. 2, 2009, pp. 315–22.

The annual premium in 2008 for an employer health plan: "Health Insurance Costs" *Fact Sheet, National Coalition on Health Care,* 2009: www.nchc.org/facts/cost.shtml.

Starbucks' chairman Howard Schultz recently noted: "Starbucks Pays More for Health Insurance Than for Coffee," A Healthy Blog, blog.hcfama.org.

A recent Harvard University study: "Illness and Injury as Contributors to Bankruptcy" by D. Himmelstein et al., Health Affairs Web Exclusive W5-63, Feb. 2, 2005; study was reported in *Health Care Costs,* National Coalition on Health Care, www.nchc.org/facts/cost.shtml.

Another study indicated that 1.5 million families lose their homes to foreclosure: Attributed to RealTruth.org in "Trickle Down Economics: Economic Crisis Seeping into Health Care Crisis" by Dustin Ensinger, *EconomyInCrisis,* Feb. 11, 2009, economyincrisis.org.

A study of Iowa consumers: "Facts on Health Care Costs," National Coalition on Health Care, www.nchc.org/documents/cost_fact_sheet_2008.pdf.

According to the Kaiser Family Foundation: The Henry J. Kaiser Family Foundation, Employee Health Benefits: 2008 Annual Survey, Sept. 2008.

[GERD] accounts for 4.6 million doctor visits each year: "Endoscopic Antireflux Procedures: A Good Wrap?" by D. Wakelin and R. Sampliner, *Clinical Gastroenterology and Hepatology* 3(9), Sept. 2005, pp. 831–39.

The Congressional Budget Office has reported: "Technological Change and the Growth of Health Care Spending," Congressional Budget Office, Jan. 2008, www.cbo.gov/ftpdocs/89xx/doc8947/01-31-TechHealth.pdf.

It is speculated that CT scans being done now will result: From Dr. Alan Bates, family physician and Oregon state senator, quoted in *Health, Money and Fear,* a documentary by Dr. Paul Hochfeld.

Even mammograms can be dangerous: "Dangers and Unreliability of Mammography: Breast Examination Is a Safe, Effective, and Practical Alternative," Cancer Prevention Coalition, www.preventcancer.com.

Reforming malpractice laws would curb defensive practices: From *Health, Money and Fear,* a documentary by Dr. Paul Hochfeld.

100 million prescriptions were written for it: "The Lessons of Vioxx — Drug Safety and Sales" by H.Waxman, *New England Journal of Medicine* 352 (25), June 2005, pp. 2576–78.

America is one of only two developed countries: "Are Direct to Consumer Drug Ads Doomed?" by Sean Gregory, *Time,* Feb. 4, 2009, www.time.com.

As Dr. John Santa . . . said recently: "Latest Medical Advance Often a Miracle That Misfires" by Joe Rojas-Burke, *The Oregonian,* Jan. 7, 2009.

Approximately 40 percent of all medical schools teach virtually nothing on the subject: "A Survey of Nutrition in Medical School Curricula" by LuAnn Soliah, *Today's Dietitian,* Feb. 2004, www.todays dietitian.com.

Specialists, who typically make far more: "Spread the Wealth Controversy Hits Doctors" by Niko Karvounis and Maggie Mahar, *Health Beat,* Nov. 14, 2008, www .healthbeatblog.org.

Ten members of this FDA panel: "10 Voters on Panel Backing Pain Pills Had Industry Ties" by G. Harris and A. Berenson, *New York Times,* Feb. 25, 2005; also "Vioxx Reapproved by FDA Panel Members with

Ties to Drug Companies," *San Francisco Chronicle,* Feb. 25, 2005.

As many as sixty thousand people may have died from taking Vioxx: "David Graham on the Vioxx Verdict" by Matthew Harper, Forbes.com, Aug. 19, 2005.

The New York Attorney General's office: "Is Industry-funded Science Killing You?" by Ronald Bailey, *Reason Online,* Oct. 2007, www.reason.com.

A recent Health and Human Services study: "HHS Report Slams FDA's Conflict of Interest Oversight" by E. Walker, *MedPage Today,* Jan.12, 2009, www.medpagetoday.com/PublicHealthPolicy/ClinicalTrials/12407. *Also:* "FDA Screening Unreliable, Study Says," Associated Press, Jan. 11, 2009.

A 2002 study of generic diuretic pills: "Major Outcomes in High-Risk Hypertensive Patients Randomized to Angiotensin-Converting Enzyme Inhibitor or Calcium Channel Blocker Vs. Diuretic; The Anti-hypertensive and Lipid-Lowering Treatment to Prevent Heart Attack Trial (ALLHAT)," written by The ALLHAT Officers and Coordinators for the ALL-HAT Collaborative Research Group, *Journal of the American Medical Association* 288(23), Dec. 15, 2002, pp. 2981–97.

As recently as the 1980s, the government funded most of the medical research on humans: From the *Journal of Pain,* cited by www.eurekalert.org, Dec. 11, 2008.

The editor of the respected British journal Lancet *recently remarked:* "For Science's Gatekeepers, a Credibility Gap" by L. Altman, M.D., *New York Times,* May 2, 2006.

Evidence-based medicine: "Evidence-based Common Sense?" by M. Sherman, *Canadian Family Physician* 54, Feb. 2008, pp. 166–68; "Parachute Use to Prevent Death and Major Trauma Related to Gravitational Challenge: Systematic Review of Randomized Controlled Trials" by G. Smith and J. Pell, *British Medical Journal* 327, Dec. 2003, pp. 1459–61.

Over a recent nine-year period the incomes of doctors: "Sources of U.S. Physician Income: The Contribution of Government Payments to the Specialist-Generalist Income Gap" by K. Lasser et al., *Journal of General Internal Medicine* 23(9), Sept. 2008, pp. 2477–81.

Chapter 3. Moving to the Future While Learning from the Past

In the 1950s:. "The 1950's: The Doctor's Office," eNotes, www.enotes.com.

That era has been called the Golden Age of

Medicine: The Rise and Fall of Modern Medicine by James Le Fanu, M.D., Carroll & Graf, New York, 1999.
We paid for routine dental and medical services out of pocket, which was common: Overdo$ed America: The Broken Promise of American Medicine* by John Abramson, Harper Perennial, New York, 2005, p. 79.
The rate of increase in the cost of health care: Consumer Price Index statistics, *Historical Statistics of the United States* (USGPO, 1975), and the annual *Statistical Abstracts of the United States,* reported in The Inflation Calculator, www.westegg.com/inflation, on rate of inflation. "Important Events in Medicine, 1950–1959," *American Decades,* E-Notes.com, *www.enotes .com/1950-medicine-health-american-decades/important-events-medicine-health,* on health-care spending in 1950, "The Rise and Rise of Healthcare Spending," *Future Healthcare,* Q 3, 2008, www.future healthcareus.com/?mc=The-Rise-and-Rise-of-Healthcare-Spending&page=miviewarticle; and "Why Does Health Care Cost So Much?" by Shannon Brownlee, *AARP Magazine,* July & Aug. 2008, www.aarpmagazine.org/health/health_care_costs.html on current health spending.

More than 70 million Americans currently have heart disease: "Vision for a Healthier America" (Sept. 2007), Trust for America's Health; healthyamericans.org/assets/files/WorkingPaper092407.pdf.

The president of the American College of Cardiology: "Heart Disease Is Still the Most Likely Reason You'll Die" by Mary Carter, CNN.com, Nov. 1, 2006 (quoting Steven Nissen, M.D.).

According to a Johns Hopkins analysis: Overdo\$ed America: The Broken Promise of American Medicine by John Abramson, Harper Perennial, New York, 2005, p. 47.

The overall death rate from cancer: "Cancer Incidence Rates Increasing" by Sharon Begley, *Wall Street Journal,* Oct. 16, 2002. "Liver Cancer Incidence Has Tripled Since 1970s, but Survival Rates Improving," *Science News,* Feb. 18, 2009. "Skin Cancer Rate Increasing" by William C. Shiel, Jr., M.D., MedicineNet.com, www.medicinenet.com/script/main/art.asp?articlekey. "Global Increase in Testicular Cancer," About.com *Men's Health,* August 6, 2006, www.menshealth.about.com. *The Politics of Cancer* by Samuel Epstein, M.D., East Ridge Press, New York, 1998, pp. 1–6. "Breast Cancer Rates Increase, but Number of Deaths Falls" by

Liz Szabo, *USA Today,* Oct. 5, 2005. "The Role of Increasing Detection in the Rising Incidence of Prostate Cancer" by A. L. Potosky et al., *Journal of the American Medical Association,* 273: 7, Feb. 15, 1995. "American Cancer Society Predicts Cancer Deaths to Increase in 2007 Despite Long Rate of Decline," *Senior Journal,* seniorjournal.com/NEWS/Health/2007/7-01-18-CancerSociety.

Cancer has overtaken heart disease as the leading cause of death: "Proportionate Mortality Trends: 1950 Through 1986," *Journal of the American Medical Association,* Dec. 26, 1990.

Chapter 4. Reversing the Toxic Trends

At least one million children, mostly boys, take Ritalin and Adderall for ADHD: "School Nurses Monitoring Children with ADHD" by Megan Flaherty, *Nurseweek,* February 8, 1999, *www.nurseweek.com/ features/99-2/ritalin.html.* Also *Healing the New Childhood Epidemics* by Kenneth Bock, M.D., and Cameron Stauth, Ballantine Books, New York, 2007, pp. 105–17. "Bridging Theory and Practice: Conceptual Understanding of Treatments for Children with Attention Deficit Hyperactivity Disorder (ADHD), Obsessive-

Compulsive Disorder (OCD), Autism, and Depression" by M. D. Rapport, M.D., *Journal of Clinical Child Psychology* 30(1), 2001, pp. 3–7.

Pharmacists fill more than 35 million prescriptions for sleep medications every year: "Americans May Be Relying Too Heavily on Sleeping Pills When Safer Remedies Are Available," *Consumer Reports,* Sept. 2006; cited on ConsumersUnion.org, www.consumersunion.org/pub/core_health_care/003660.html.

An estimated 81 percent of all Americans take at least one prescribed medication every day: "Why Americans Take So Many Prescription Drugs" by J. Douglas Bremmer, M.D., www.oftwominds.com.

A recent report from the U.S. Centers for Disease Control and Prevention showed: "Ten Great Public Health Achievements — United States, 1900–1999," *Morbidity and Mortality Weekly Report,* April 2, 1999, cited in "Public Health Institutes and Health Change Strategies" by Jeffrey R. Taylor, Ph.D., Michigan Public Health Institute, Oct. 2005, www.mphi.org.

Another recent study, published in the American Journal of Public Health: "A Hurdle for Health Reform: Patients and Their Doctors" by T. Parker-Pope, *New York*

Times News Service, Jan. 2009, citing "The Health Impact of Resolving Racial Disparities: An Analysis of U.S. Mortality Data" by S. Woolf et al., *American Journal of Public Health* 94(12), Dec. 2004, pp. 2078–81.

David Newman, M.D., stressed: "A Hurdle for Health Reform: Patients and Their Doctors" by T. Parker-Pope, *New York Times,* Mar. 2, 2009.

In Scandinavia, Germany, France, the United Kingdom, and Canada: Critical — What We Can Do About the Health-Care Crisis by Senator Tom Daschle, with Scott S. Greenberger and Jeanne M. Lambrew, Thomas Dunne Books, St. Martin's Press, New York, 2008.

The high costs of American medicine . . . also put American business at a great disadvantage globally: A Second Opinion — Rescuing America's Health Care by Arnold S. Relman, M.D., A Century Foundation Book, Public Affairs, New York, 2007.

Harvard business professor Regina Herzlinger has examined: Who Killed Health Care? America's $2 Trillion Medical Problem — and the Consumer-Driven Cure by Regina Herzlinger, McGraw-Hill, New York, 2007, p. 103.

One hospital in Bangkok, Thailand: Critical:

What We Can Do About the Health-Care Crisis by Tom Daschle (with Scott S. Greenberger and Jeanne M. Lambrew), Thomas Dunne Books, St. Martin's Press, New York, 2008, p. 13.

Labor unions fought a national health insurance plan: One Nation Uninsured: Why the U.S. Has No National Health Insurance by Jill Quadagno, Oxford University Press, New York, 2005. (Other sources: www .spectator.org, www.healthcare.change .org/blog, www.enotes.com.)

The American Medical Association . . . fought tooth and nail against it: Ibid.

Annual surveys by the Massachusetts Medical Society: Berkshire Eagle, Pittsfield, Mass., Oct. 24, 2007.

Clem Whitaker . . . said: One Nation Uninsured: Why the U.S. Has No National Health Insurance by Jill Quadagno, Oxford University Press, New York, 2005, p. 35.

Robert Taft . . . blasted Truman's plan: The Social Transformation of American Medicine by Paul Starr, Basic Books, New York, 1984, p. 283.

Rudolph Giuliani said: "Giuliani Attacks Democrats Health Plans as Socialist" by Paul Steinhauser, CNN Politics.com, Aug. 1, 2007, www.politicalticker.blogs.cnn .com.

Arnold Relman, M.D., coined the phrase *"medical industrial complex"*: "Shift Happens: Why Is America's Health-Care System Collapsing? Three Books, Three Good Answers" by Jerry Avorn, *The American Prospect,* Oct. 30, 2007; referring to the phrase's first appearance in Relman's article "The New Medical-Industrial Complex" in the *New England Journal of Medicine* 303, 1980, pp. 963–70.

The Cost of American Health Care: This was calculated from numerous sources, among them the U.S. Bureau of the Census, *Statistical Abstract of the U.S.: 1989* (Washington, D.C., U.S. Government Printing Office, 1989), enotes.com, The National Coalition on Health Care (www.nchc.org/facts/cost.shtml), and the Kaiser Family Foundation (www.kff.org).

One recent study showed that patients routinely demand unnecessary drugs: "Burden of Difficult Encounters in Primary Care: Data from the Minimizing Error, Maximizing Outcomes Study" by P. An et al. for the MEMO Investigators, *Archives of Internal Medicine* 169(4), 2009, pp. 410–14. Reported in "A Hurdle for Health Reform — Patients and Their Doctors" by T. Parker-Pope, *New York Times,* Mar.

2, 2009.

Dr. Marcia Angell . . . recently noted: "A Hurdle for Health Reform" by T. Parker Pope, *New York Times,* Mar. 2, 2009.

Medical scanning has become a $100-billion-per year business and *Bruce Hillman, M.D., said:* "Good or Useless, Medical Scans Cost the Same," *New York Times,* nytimes.com, Mar. 2, 2009.

Hospitals are America's largest single driver of health-care costs: "Technological Change and the Growth of Health Care Spending," Congressional Budget Office Paper, Jan. 2008 (2005 dollars), p. 6.

For-profit hospitals, according to a 2002 study, had a 2 percent higher risk of patient death: "A Systematic Review and Meta-Analysis of Studies Comparing Mortality Between Private For-Profit and Private Not-For-Profit Hospitals" by P. Devereaux et al., *Canadian Medical Association Journal* 166(11), May 28, 2002, pp. 1399–1406.

A 2009 Dartmouth study: "Slowing the Growth of Health Care Costs — Lessons from Regional Variation" by E. Fisher et al., *New England Journal of Medicine,* 360(9), Feb. 2009, pp. 849–52.

The health insurance industry rakes in staggering profits: "Top Industries: Most Profitable," Fortune 500, *Fortune,* May 5,

2008; April 30, 2007; money.cnn.com; Fortune Global 500 in *Fortune,* July 23, 2007, as cited on CNNMoney.com (money.cnn.com/magazines/fortune/global500/2007/industries/223/1.html); *Forbes,* www.forbes.com/static/pvp2005/LIRRI3M.html; "Options Scandal Claims UnitedHealth's McGuire" by Scott Reeves, Forbes.com, Oct. 16, 2006 (www.forbes.com/2006/10/16/mcguire-unitedhealth-options-face-cx_sr_1016 autofacescan02.html); Health Care for America Now (healthcare foramericanow .org/site/content/10_questions_to_ ask_a hip_about_their_health_care_reform_pro posal).

By the 1960s more than seven hundred companies were selling health insurance in the United States and raking in lots of money: Health Care Crisis, PBS Health — Timeline — www.pbs.org/healthcare crisis/history.htm.

President Nixon was convinced by a Minnesota doctor: The Health Care Mess: How We Got into It and How We'll Get Out of It by Kip Sullivan, AuthorHouse, Bloomington, Ind., 2006. Another source: *Critical Condition: How Health Care in America Became Big Business — and Bad Medicine* by Donald L. Barlett and James B. Steele,

Broadway Books, New York, 2006.

A taped conversation: Who Killed Health Care? America's $2 Trillion Medical Problem — and the Consumer-Driven Cure by Regina Herzlinger, McGraw-Hill, New York, 2007, pp. 108–9.

Chapter 5. Doctors of the Future

Thomas Edison who spoke those words: "Doctor of the Future," www.snopes.com, quoting from 1902 article, "Edison Hails Era of Speed," *Fort Wayne Sentinel,* Dec. 31, 1902, p. 49.

Too many patients describe their doctors as not being "people persons": "Joint Commission Issues Rules Designed to Stop Bad Behavior by Doctors" by Anne Zieger, July 10, 2008, www.fiercehealth care.com.

The Mayo Clinic recently did a patient survey: "7 Key Traits of the Ideal Doctor" by N. Bendapudi, *Mayo Clinic Proceedings* 81, Mar. 2006, pp. 338–44.

The $1-billion-per-year antidepressant drug Paxil: "Glaxo Attracts Questions on Data in Paxil Studies," *Wall Street Journal,* Jun. 14, 2008; online.wsj.com/article/ SB121339980355773595.html?mod=goo glenews_wsj.

A Harvard psychiatrist reported recently that

patients on Paxil: *Prozac Backlash: Overcoming the Dangers of Prozac, Zoloft, Paxil, and Other Antidepressants with Safe, Effective Alternatives* by Joseph Glenmullen, M.D., Touchstone, Beaverton, Ore., 2000, pp. 135–89.

Between 1997 and 2005, the number of doctors who became primary care physicians: Physicians Index, July 8, 2008, www.salon.com.

Only 31 percent of all American doctors are in primary care: Medscape, www.medscape.com. Statistic confirmed in *Rx for Health Care Reform* by Ken Terry, Vanderbilt University Press, Nashville, Tenn., 2007, p. 170.

A recent study showed that the states in America with the highest ratio of primary care doctors: Health Policy: Crisis and Reform in the U.S. Health Care Delivery System by Charlene Harrington et al., Jones & Bartlett Publishers, Sudbury, Mass., 2004, p. 49; citing "Income Inequality, Primary Care, and Health Indicators" by L. Shi et al., *Journal of Family Practice,* 48(4), Apr. 1999, pp. 275–84.

According to the Bureau of Labor Statistics: "Earnings of Primary Care Physicians" by Laurence Shatkin, *Fast Company,* Oct. 29, 2008, fastcompany.com.

Martin J. Blaser, M.D. . . . has commented: www.news-medical.net/print_article.asp?id=24007.

Physicist Steven Hawking, Ph.D., once said: Complexity Explained by Peter Erdi, Springer, 2007, p. 1, quoting Hawking in *Complexity Digest* 10, Mar. 5, 2001.

A recent study showed that brevity of doctor visits: "Diversifying the Options for Interacting with Patients," *Quality and Safety in Health Care* 6, no. 5, p. 322.

Hawaii recently became the first state: "Hawaii Tries Out Online Health Care" by Ina Fried, *Cutting Edge,* CNET News, Jan. 15, 2009, www.news.cnet.com.

E-visit: "Call Your Doctor Online: The Medicine of the Future?" by Bertalan Mesko, *Science Roll,* May 18, 2005, scienceroll.com.

Roy Schoenberg . . . has said: "Hawaii Tries Out Online Health Care" by Ina Fried, *Cutting Edge,* CNET News, Jan. 15, 2009, www.news.cnet.com.

Remote monitoring: "Remote Healthcare Monitoring Not So Distant," *Medical News Today,* www.medicalnewstoday.com.

A recent report by Pew Research: "Internet Use Among College Students for Health Related Information," PHI Wiki Project, www.phiwiki.wetpaint.com.

President Barack Obama has proposed spending $50 billion: "The Evidence Gap; Health Care That Puts a Computer on the Team" by Steve Lohr, *New York Times,* Jan. 16, 2009.

Only about 20 percent of all doctors now use electronic records: "On the Front Lines of Care: Primary Care Doctors Office Systems, Experiences, and Views in Seven Countries" by Cathy Schoen et al., Nov. 2, 2006, www.commonwealthfund.org. *Also:* "Wal-Mart to Enter Electronic Medical Records Arena," Associated Press, Mar. 11, 2009.

Between 2005 and 2009, insurance and pharmaceutical companies donated: "Health Sector Has Donated Millions to Lawmakers" by Dan Eggen, *Washington Post,* Mar. 9, 2009.

The biggest beneficiaries: "Will Baucus' HMO and Drug Company Bucks Foil Obamacare?" by Jamie Court, *Consumer Watchdog,* www.consumerwatchdog.org. *Also:* "Senators Who Weakened Drug Bill Got Millions from Industry" by Ken Dilanian, *USA Today,* www.usatoday.com, May 11, 2007.

A recent New York Times *article:* "Harvard Medical School in Ethics Quandary," *New York Times,* Mar. 3, 2009.

In 2008 Harvard accepted almost $12 million from drug companies: Ibid.

"The Healer's Art": "The Healer's Art," Oregon CAM Course at OHSU (Oregon Health Sciences University), www.ohsu.edu.

Chapter 6. Medicine of the Future

Robert Fulford: Dr. Fulford's Touch of Life by Robert Fulford, D.O., Pocket Books, New York, 1970.

An estimated 36 percent of Americans receive a professional massage: "2008 Massage Therapy Consumer Survey Fact Sheet," American Massage Therapy Association, www.amtamassage.org.

Qingcai Zhang, M.D.: www.sinomedresearch.org/drz.htm.

Acupuncture can produce dramatic improvement: www.essentialhealthcare.com/info_for_practitioners/efficacy.html.

My long experience with botanical medicine: Health and Healing by Andrew Weil, M.D., Houghton Mifflin, Boston, rev. ed., 1998, pp. 96–111.

One pioneer of this research, Richard Davidson, Ph.D.: "Meditation, Positive Emotions and Brain Science" by Richard Davidson, interviewed by Daniel Redwood, HealthWorld Online, 2007, www.healthy.net.

As many as 70 percent of all visits to family doctors are for stress-related disorders: "Stress Management for Patient and Physician," www.mentalhealth.com.

Obesity: "Chronic Obesity — Preventing Obesity and Chronic Diseases Through Good Nutrition and Physical Activity," Centers for Disease Control and Prevention, www.cdc.gov.

Inappropriate inflammation: Healthy Aging by Andrew Weil, M.D., Anchor Books, Random House, New York, 2005, pp. 170–96.

Dietary Supplementation: Ibid., pp. 197–216. *Also:* "Antioxidants and Cancer Prevention: Fact Sheet," National Cancer Institute, www.cancer.gov.

As recently as the early 1900s, most people in America: Brain Longevity by Dharma Singh Kahlsa, M.D., and Cameron Stauth, Warner Books, New York, 1997, p. 326.

Exercise . . . has innumerable beneficial effects: One Body, One Life by Gregory Joujon-Roche and Cameron Stauth, Dutton, New York, 2006, pp. 69–71.

Chapter 7. The New American Health Care
Adverse drug reactions account for a great deal of unnecessary illness and death: "Incidence of Adverse Drug Reactions in

371

Hospitalized Patients: A Meta-Analysis of Prospective Studies" by J. Lazarou et al., *Journal of the American Medical Association* 279, 1998, pp. 1200–1205.

One study of drug brochures given to doctors: "Data in Drug Promotional Brochures Can Be Inaccurate," *ScienceDaily,* March 4, 2006, www.sciencedaily.com.

The pharmaceutical industry reaps egregious profits: The Truth About the Drug Companies: How They Deceive Us and What to Do About It by Marcia Angell, Random House, New York, 2005.

Said . . . Dr. Catherine DeAngelis: "Impugning the Integrity of Medical Science: The Adverse Effects of Industry" by C. DeAngelis and P. Fontanarosa, *Journal of the American Medical Association* 299(15), Apr. 2008, pp. 1833–35.

They spent $138 million in 2007: "Health Care Industry Spent $445 Million on Federal Lobbying in 2007," *Kaiser Daily Health Policy Report,* April 15, 2008, www.kaisernetwork.org/Daily_Reports/print_report.cfm?DR_ID=51546&dr_cat=3.

Americans are now exposed to seven times as much cancer-causing radiation as they were in 1980: "Overexposed: Imaging Tests Boost U.S. Radiation Dose" by Julie Steenhuysen, *Reuters,* Mar. 3, 2009, www

.reuters.com.

Chapter 8. Disease Prevention: The Sustainable Solution

Chronic diseases cause 70 percent of deaths in America: "Vision for a Healthier America," Trust for America's Health, Sept. 2007, healthyamericans.org.

One study showed that women who maintain a healthy weight: "Obesity, Diet and Risk of Non-Hodgkin Lymphoma" by C. Skibola, *Cancer Epidemiology Biomarkers & Prevention* 16, Mar, 1, 2007, p. 392.

Laughter can turn off some of the genes that control the expression of type-2 diabetes: "Laughter Regulates Gene Expression in Patients with Type-2 Diabetes" by T. Hayashi et al., *Psychotherapy and Psychosomatics* 75(1), 2006, pp. 62–65.

The CDC estimates that each year 1.7 million Americans die: Testimony by Julie Gerberding, director of Centers for Disease Control and Prevention, Department of Health and Human Services, on the CDC's Role in Promoting Healthy Lifestyles, before the Senate Committee on Appropriations, Subcommittee on Labor, HHS, Education and Related Agencies, Jan. 17, 2003.

A recent study reported in the New England

Journal of Medicine: "A Potential Decline in Life Expectancy in the United States in the 21st Century" by S. Jay Olshansky et al., *New England Journal of Medicine* 352(11), Mar. 17, 2005, pp. 1138–45.

As Harvard's Walter Willett, M.D., recently noted: "Teaching Doctors to Teach Patients About Lifestyle" by Kate Murphy, *New York Times,* Apr. 17, 2007.

Almost 40 percent of American hospitals have fast-food restaurants on their premises: "Marketing Fast Food: Impact of Fast Food Restaurants in Children's Hospitals" by H. Sahud et al., *Pediatrics* 118(6), Dec. 2006, pp. 2290–97. The article cites a *U.S. News & World Report* "Honor Roll" of hospitals — America's best, in their evaluation — from 2001; 38 percent of these had fast-food restaurants on their premises.

Only 11 percent of Americans meet the USDA guidelines: "Have Americans Increased Their Fruit and Vegetable Intake? The Trends Between 1988 and 2002" by S. Stark et al., *American Journal of Preventive Medicine* 32(4), Apr. 2007, pp. 257–63.

Studies indicate that a diet high in fruits and vegetables: "Blood Pressure and Vitamin C and Fruit and Vegetable Intake" by R. Beitz et al., *Annals of Nutritional Metabo-*

lism 47, 2003, pp. 214–20.

Many fruits and vegetables contain phyto-nutrients: "Phytonutrients: A More Natural Approach Toward Cancer Prevention" by S. D'Ambrosio, *Seminars in Cancer Biology* 17 (5), Oct. 2007, pp. 345–46.

A diet rich in the flavonoids: "Flavonoid Intake and Colorectal Cancer Risk in Men and Women" by J. Lin et al., *American Journal of Epidemiology* 164(7), 2006, pp. 644–51.

Cruciferous vegetables: "Diet, GSTM1 and GSTT1 and Head and Neck Cancer" by M. Gaudet et al., *Carcinogenesis* 25(5), May 2004, pp. 735–40.

Compounds in onions and garlic: "Allium Vegetables and Organosulfur Compounds: Do They Help Prevent Cancer?" by F. Bianchini and H. Vainio, *Environmental Health Perspectives* 109(9), Sept. 2001, pp. 893–902.

The phytoestrogens in soy appear to lower the incidence: "Soy Intake and Cancer Risk: A Review of the In Vitro and In Vivo Data" by F. Sarkar and Y. Li, *Cancer Investigation* 21(5), 2003, pp. 744–57.

Most cases of type-2 diabetes can be successfully controlled: "Systematic Review of Herbs and Dietary Supplements for Glycemic Control in Diabetes" by G. Yeh et al., *Diabetes Care* 26(4), 2003, pp. 1277–94.

The nutrient lutein: "The Relationship of Dietary Carotenoid and Vitamin A, E, and C Intake with Age-Related Macular Degeneration in a Case-Controlled Study" by AREDS research group, *Archives of Ophthalmology* 125(9), Sept. 2007, pp. 1225–32.

The B-complex of vitamins has a number of preventive properties: "Mortality and Cardiovascular Events in Patients Treated with Homocysteine-Lowering B Vitamins After Coronary Angiography," *Journal of the American Medical Association* 300 (7), Aug. 20, 2008, pp. 795–804; "Consensus Paper on the Rational Clinical Use of Homocysteine, Folic Acid and B Vitamins in Cardiovascular and Thrombotic Diseases: Guidelines and Recommendations," *Clinical Chemistry and Laboratory Medicine* 41 (11), Nov. 2003, pp. 1392–1403. "The Vitamin B Complex and Functional Chronic Gastro-Intestinal Malfunction: A Study of Two Hundred and Twenty-seven Cases," *American Journal of Digestive Diseases* 5(4), Apr. 1938.

Selenium may significantly reduce the risk of

prostate cancer: "Selenium Supplementation, Baseline Plasma Selenium Status and Incidence of Prostate Cancer: An Analysis of the Complete Treatment Period of the Nutritional Prevention of Cancer Trial" by A. Duffield-Lillico et al., *British Journal of Urology International* 91(7), Apr. 2003, pp. 608–12.

Vitamin C has a wide range of preventive actions: "Might Vitamin C Prevent Gout?" The C.A.M. Report, www.thecamreport .com; "Can Vitamin C Prevent Ulcers?" DrWeil.Com, www.drweil.com; "Vitamin C Prevents Pregnancy Complication," www.ambafrance-do.org. "Vitamin C Prevents Cancer by Blocking Hydrogen Peroxide, but Apple Chemical Works Even Better, Cornell and Korean Scientists Report," www.news.cornell.edu, Jan. 21, 2002.

Vitamin D is vital to proper immune function: The UV Advantage: The Medical Breakthrough That Shows How to Harness the Power of the Sun for Your Health by Michael F. Holick, IBooks, New York, 2007. *Also:* "Vitamin D: Importance in the Prevention of Cancers, Type 1 Diabetes, Heart Disease, and Osteoporosis" by Michael F. Holick, *American Journal of Clinical Nutrition* 80 (suppl.), Mar. 2004, pp.

1678S–88S.

Preventive Benefits of Exercise: "Girls, Young Women Can Cut Risk of Early Breast Cancer Through Regular Exercise," *Science Daily,* May 14, 2008, reporting a joint study by Washington University School of Medicine and Harvard University; "Exercises Can Ease Arthritis Pain" by Dr. Richard Weil, WebMD, www.webmd.com. "The Effects of Exercise on Cancer to Be Studied with $7 Million Grant," Yale School of Public Health, March 23, 2009, www.healthnewsdigest.com. "Exercise Effects on Depressive Symptoms and Self-worth in Overweight Children: A Randomized Controlled Trial" by K. Petty et al., *Journal of Pediatric Psychology Advance Access,* published online, Feb. 16, 2009.

Preventive Benefits of Stress Management: "Meditation, Breath Work, and Focus Training for Teachers and Students — Five Minutes a Day That Can Really Make a Difference" by Sandra A. Sessa, *Journal of College Teaching & Learning,* Oct. 2007; *Brain Longevity* by Dharma Singh Khalsa, M.D., and Cameron Stauth, Warner Books, New York, 1997.

Sleeping fewer than seven hours per night has been shown to increase the risk: "Sleep Habits and Susceptibility to the Common

Cold" by S. Cohen et al., *Archives of Internal Medicine* 169(1), 2009, pp. 62–67; *also:* healthysleep.med.harvard.edu/healthy/matters/consequences/sleep-and-disease-risk.

The Toll of Smoking: "Smoking Is a Risk Factor for Multiple Sclerosis" by T. Riise et al., *Neurology* 61, Oct. 2003, pp. 1122–24; "Cigarette Smoking and Age-Related Macular Degeneration in the EUREYE Study" by U. Chakravarthy et al., *Ophthalmology,* 114, 2007, pp. 1157–63; "Smoking-Attributable Mortality, Years of Potential Life Lost, and Productivity Losses, United States, 2000–2004," *Morbidity and Mortality Weekly Report* 57(45), 2008, pp. 1226–28; "Levels of Excess Infant Deaths Attributable to Maternal Smoking During Pregnancy in the United States" by H. Salihu et al., *Maternal and Child Health Journal* 7(4), Dec. 2003, pp. 219–27; "The Causal Role of Cigarette Smoking in Bladder Cancer Initiation and Progression, and the Role of Urologists in Smoking Cessation," *Journal of Urology* 180, July 2008, pp. 31–37.

Not until the mid-1980s did the American Medical Association: "Tobacco Divestment and Fiduciary Responsibility: A Legal and

Financial Analysis, 2000," Employee Benefits Legal Resource Site, Jan. 15, 2000, benefitsattorney.com/modules.php ?name=Reviews&rop=showcontent&id=3.

Analysts have tried to evaluate the effect that each of these antismoking strategies has had: "Smoking and Public Policy," *Encyclopedia Britannica,* www.britannica.com/ EBchecked/topic/550049/smoking/ 242786/Smoking-and-public-policy. *Also:* "Tobacco Control Factsheets, Tobacco-Control Resource Center and the International Union Against Cancer, www.globalink .org/en/advertising.shtml.

In Pueblo, Colorado, for example, a ban on public smoking: "Dramatic Drop in Heart Attacks Attributed to Smoking Ban" by Madeline Ellis, *HealthNews,* Jan. 3, 2009, www.healthnews.com/family-health/ dramatic-drop-heart-attacks-attributed-smoking-ban-2385.html.

The Walgreen Company . . . has asked a California state court: http://abclocal.go.com/ kgo/story?section=news/local&id=6380 311.

Car wrecks kill about 42,000 people each year: "Traffic Safety Facts," National Highway Traffic Safety Administration (2006 figure).

The disorder is called metabolic syndrome:

Metabolic Syndrome and Cardiovascular Disease by T. Barry Levine and Arlene Bradley Levine, Saunders, New York, 2006; *The Metabolic Syndrome Program: How to Lose Weight, Beat Heart Disease, Stop Insulin Resistance, and More* by Karlene Karst, Wiley, New York, 2006.

The Toll of Obesity: "Obesity Strongest Risk Factor for Colorectal Cancer," from a report by the American College of Gastroenterology, *Science Daily,* Oct. 15, 2007. "First Sister Study Results Reinforce the Importance of Healthy Living," *Science Daily,* Mar. 16, 2009, www.cdc.gov. "Prepregnancy and Obesity" by Doug Brunk, www.mdconsult.com. "Overweight/Obesity 'Enormous' Risk Factor for ESRD — End Stage Renal Disease" by Caroline Cassels, Medscape, Jan. 9, 2006, based on an article in *Annals of Internal Medicine,* Jan. 3, 2006, www.medscape.com. "Is Obesity a Risk Factor for Cancer?" *Journal of Allergy and Clinical Immunology* 115(5), May 2005, pp. 925–27; *also:* www.obesity.org, Web site of The Obesity Society.

The Farm Bill: Food Fight: The Citizen's Guide to a Food and Farm Bill by Daniel Imhoff and Michael Pollan, University of California Press, Berkeley, Calif., 2007.

In July 2008 the Los Angeles City Council

voted unanimously: "LA Blocks New Fast-Food Outlets from Poor Areas" by Christina Hoag, Associated Press, July 28, 2008.

American College of Preventive Medicine: www.acpm.org.

The sunscreen industry: www.sunlightscam .com/aad.html. *Also:* www.doctoryourself .com/holick.html.

Elevated serum cholesterol: What Your Doctor May Not Tell You About Cholesterol by Stephen R. Devries and Winifred Conkling, Wellness Centrasl (Hachette), Boston, 2007.

A manufacturer-sponsored study addressed the benefit of 10 milligrams daily of Lipitor: "Prevention of Coronary and Stroke Events with Atorvastatin in Hypertensive Patients Who Have Average or Lower-Than-Average Cholesterol Concentrations, in the Anglo-Scandinavian Cardiac Outcomes Trial — Lipid Lowering Arm (ASCOT-LLA): A Multicentre Randomized Controlled Trial" by P. S. Sever et al., *Lancet* 361(9364), 2003, pp. 1149–58; *also,* www.medicine.ox.ac.uk/bandolier/ band47/b47-2.html#Heading7.

[Lipitor], like other statins . . . can cause adverse effects: www.sciencedaily.com/ releases/2009/01/090127090735.htm.

Bisphosphonates are not benign: www.webmd

.com/osteoporosis/bisphosphonates-for-osteoporosis.

An excerpt from information for doctors on Fosamax: https://www.fosamax.com.sa/secure/about/about_fosamax.html.

Even more recent research suggests that consuming more folate: "Folate Fortification: Enough Already?" by Barry Shane, *American Journal of Clinical Nutrition* 77(1), Jan. 2000, pp. 8–9.

X-rays and CT scans: "When X-ray, MRI and CT Scans Harm More Than Help" by Joe Rojas-Burke, *The Oregonian,* Feb. 18, 2009.

Chapter 9. Health Promotion: The Critical Component

In Japan health officials measure the waistlines of people over forty: "Japan, Seeking Trim Waists, Measures Millions" by Norimitsu Onishi, *New York Times,* June 13, 2008.

New Zealand even has a rule that bars obese people from immigrating to the country: "Obese Migrant Told to Lose Weight Before Making Move" by Kathy Marks, *The Independent,* www.independent.co.uk, Nov. 17, 2007.

Nanny State: How Food Fascists, Teetotaling Do-Gooders, Priggish Moralists, and Other

Boneheaded Bureaucrats Are Turning America into a Nation of Children by Daniel Harsanyi, Broadway, New York, 2007.
A recent survey in the United Kingdom: news.bbc.co.uk/2/hi/health/3839447.stm.
Results of a survey of American health literacy: www.health.gov/communication/literacy/quickguide/factsliteracy.htm. *Also:* "Health Literacy: A Challenge for American Patients and Their Health Care Providers" by Ruth Parker, *Health Promotion International,* (15) 4, Dec. 2000, pp. 277–83, www.heapro.oxfordjournals.org.
Placebo effects are pure healing responses: Health and Healing by Andrew Weil, M.D., pp. 206–18; "The Healing Power of Placebos," *FDA Consumer* magazine, Jan./Feb. 2000; www.fda.gov. "Placebo Effect: A Cure in the Mind" by Niemi Maj-Britt, *Scientific American,* Feb. 2009. sciam.com.
Debra A. Lieberman wrote: Health Promotion and Interactive Technology: Theoretical Applications and Future Directions by Richard L. Street et al., Lawrence Erlbaum Associates, Mahway, N.J., 1997, p. 103. *Also:* "Medical Games," medicaleducation.wet paint.com.
Immune Attack: "Scientists Release Educational Computer Games" by Meris Stansbury, *eSchool News,* eschoolnews.com,

May 22, 2008.

The American Public Health Association: www.apha.org.

The CDC's mission . . . and its goals: www.cdc.gov/osi/goals/.

In July 2008 former CDC director Julie Gerberding announced: "CDC Campaign Hopes to Make USA a Healthier Nation" by Rita Rubin, *USA Today,* July 7, 2008, www.usatoday.com/news/health/2008-07-07-cdc-gerberding_N.htm.

CDC's allocation of funds: Department of Health and Human Services, Fiscal Year 2007: Centers for Disease Control and Prevention; FY 2007 CDC/ATSDR Functional Table.

In August 2008 the FDA aligned itself with the chemical industry: "FDA Decision on Safety of BPA 'Flawed' " by Liz Szabo, *USA Today,* Nov. 1, 2008, www.usatoday.com.

National Institute of Environmental Health Sciences: www.niehs.nih.gov/.

Our hospitals and medical centers are some of the worst polluters: "America's Best Hospitals, Green Edition" by Maura Judkis, *US News & World Report,* July 16, 2008, www.usnews.com/blogs; "Hospitals Among Top Polluters," *The Missoulian,* Oct. 10, 2008, www.missoulian.com/

articles/2008/10/18/news/local/news04.txt.

Germany, for one, is starting a $47 million program: "How Other Countries Fight Fat," *Parade,* Feb. 15, 2009, www.parade .com/news/intelligence-report/archive/ how-other-countries-fight-fat.html.

Banning fast-food advertising to children could reduce the number of overweight kids: "Fast-Food Restaurant Advertising on Television and Its Influence on Childhood Obesity" by Shin-Yi Chou et al., *Journal of Law and Economics* 51(4), Nov. 2008, pp. 519–618.

Kids and adults are more sedentary than ever: "Physical Activity and Health," a Report of the Surgeon General, from the National Center for Chronic Diseases Prevention and Health Promotion; www.cdc.gov; "2008 Physical Activity Guidelines for Americans," U.S. Department of Health and Human Services, www.health.gov/ paguidelines.

In July 2008 the State of Alabama announced: From the National Conference of State Legislatures; www.ncsl.org/programs/ health/stateemploy.htm.

The need for omega-3 fatty acids: "Neurodevelopmental Outcomes of Preterm Infants Fed High-Dose Docosahexaenoic Acid: A Randomized Controlled Trial" by

M. Makrides et al., *Journal of the American Medical Association* 301(2), Jan. 14, 2009, pp. 175–82.

Deficiency of DHA . . . may predispose a child to neurological, mental, and emotional problems: "Role of Docosahexaenoic Acid in Maternal and Child Mental Health" by N. Ramakrishnan et al., *American Journal of Clinical Nutrition* 89(3): Mar. 2009, pp. 958S–62S.

Chapter 10. What the Future Will Look Like

A professor of medicine at the University of California, Davis, wrote recently: "Inside Medicine: Rationed Care Creates Ethical Quandary" by Dr. Michael Wilkes, *The Sacramento Bee,* July 20, 2008, p. 1L.

Money now wasted inexcusably in administrative costs: "Why Does U.S. Health Care Cost So Much? (Part II: Indefensible Administrative Costs)" by Uwe E. Reinhardt, *New York Times,* Nov. 21, 2008, www.economix.blogs.nytimes.com.

National Summit on Obesity: www.time .com/time/health/article/0,8599,646304, 00.html.

An editorial by Drs. James Dalen and Joseph Alpert: "National Health Insurance: Could It Work in the US?" *American Journal of*

Medicine 121(7), July 2008.

The Australian health-care system is in much less trouble than ours: "World Health Organization Assesses the World's Health Systems," *The World Health Report,* 2000, The World Health Organization, www.who.int/whr/2000/media_centre/ press_release/en/index.html; "The World Health Organization's Ranking of the World's Health Systems," *WHO World Health Report,* World Health Organization press release, Feb. 28, 2007, www.photius .com/rankings/healthranks.html.

Today about 47 million Americans receive no *guarantee of basic health care:* "Census Bureau: Number of U.S. Uninsured Rises to 47 Million Americans" by Teddi D. Johnson, *Nation's Health,* Jan. 8, 2008, www.medscape.com/viewarticle/567737.

ABOUT THE AUTHOR

Andrew Weil, M.D., is the author of eleven previous books, including *Spontaneous Healing, 8 Weeks to Optimum Health,* and *Healthy Aging.* A graduate of Harvard Medical School, he is a professor of public health and a clinical professor of medicine at the University of Arizona, as well as the director of the Arizona Center for Integrative Medicine. He writes *Self Healing,* a monthly newsletter, and maintains the Web site Dr Weil.com. He lives in Arizona.

To learn more, visit:

www.drweil.com
www.whyourhealthmatters.com
www.weilfoundation.org

THE WEIL FOUNDATION

The Weil Foundation supports the advancement of integrative medicine through training, research, the education of the public, and policy reform.
**To learn more, visit
www.weilfoundation.org**

The employees of Thorndike Press hope you have enjoyed this Large Print book. All our Thorndike, Wheeler, and Kennebec Large Print titles are designed for easy reading, and all our books are made to last. Other Thorndike Press Large Print books are available at your library, through selected bookstores, or directly from us.

For information about titles, please call:
(800) 223-1244

or visit our Web site at:
http://gale.cengage.com/thorndike

To share your comments, please write:
Publisher
Thorndike Press
295 Kennedy Memorial Drive
Waterville, ME 04901